Innovations *in* Occupational Therapy Education

1999

Patricia A. Crist, PhD, OTR/L, FAOTA
Editor

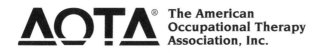

The American Occupational Therapy Association, Inc.

The American Occupational Therapy Association, Inc.
4720 Montgomery Lane
PO Box 31220
Bethesda, Maryland 20824-1220

Disclaimers

This publication is designed to provide accurate and authoritative information in regard to the subject matter covered. It is sold or distributed with the understanding that the publisher is not engaged in rendering legal, accounting, or other professional service. If legal advice or other expert assistance is required, the services of a competent professional person should be sought.
    —*From the Declaration of Principles jointly adopted by the American Bar Association and a Committee of Publishers and Associations.*

It is the objective of The American Occupational Therapy Association to be a forum for free expression and interchange of ideas. The opinions expressed by the contributors to this work are their own and not necessarily those of either the editors or The American Occupational Therapy Association.

ISBN 1-56900-119-7

Printed in the United States of America.

Table of Contents

Board Appointments

Name	Appointment
Alfred G. Bracciano, EdD, OTR	2 Year (1998–2000)
Caroline Robinson Brayley, PhD, OTR/L, FAOTA	2 Year (1998–2000)
Vera-Jean Clark-Brown, MS, L/OTR	2 Year (1998–2000)
Cynthia L. Creighton, MA, OTR/L	2 Year (1998–2000)
Nancy Lee Hollins, MS, OTR	2 Year (1998–2000)
Aimee J. Luebben, EdD, OTR/L, FAOTA	2 Year (1998–2000)
Anne Cronin Mosey, PhD, OTR, FAOTA	2 Year (1998–2000)
Annette M. Port, COTA	2 Year (1998–2000)
Wendy Starnes, OTR/L	2 Year (1998–2000)
Perri Stern, EdD, OTR	2 Year (1998–2000)
Ellen S. Cohn, EdM, OTR/L, FAOTA	3 Year (1998–2001)
Teru A. Creel, MS, OTR/L	3 Year (1998–2001)
Nedra P. Gillette, MEd, OTR, FAOTA	3 Year (1998–2001)
Caryn R. Johnson, MS, OTR/L, FAOTA	3 Year (1998–2001)
Scott D. McPhee, MS, MPA, DrPH, OTR, FAOTA	3 Year (1998–2001)
Susan Cook Merrill, MA, OTR/L	3 Year (1998–2001)
Shirley Peganoff O'Brien, MS, OTR/L, FAOTA	3 Year (1998–2001)
Peggy Owens, MA, OTR/L, FAOTA	3 Year (1998–2001)
Barbara A. Schell, PhD, OT, FAOTA	3 Year (1998–2001)
Janette K. Schkade, PhD, OTR, FAOTA	3 Year (1998–2001)
Mary P. Taugher, PhD, FAOTA	3 Year (1998–2001)
Louise R. Thibodaux, MA, OTR/L, FAOTA	3 Year (1998–2001)
Kay F. Walker, PhD, FAOTA	3 Year (1998–2001)

Editor
| Patricia A. Crist, PhD, OTR/L, FAOTA | 3 Year (1998–2001) |

Innovation to Action

Karen Jacobs

We live in uncertain and unpredictable times, which makes educating future occupational therapy practitioners even more of a challenge. The rigor required to become a competent, ethical, and skilled practitioner seems to increase daily, as we face an ever changing, complex health care environment and evolving occupational therapy theories and models that support evidence-based outcomes. The great challenge we face as occupational therapy educators is: What is the best way to prepare occupational therapy students to successfully meet the challenges of the future? I answer this question not as a prognosticator, but rather as an educator who is involved in all levels of education (academia, clinical practice, and continuing education). I believe we can begin by being role models or mentors to our students by imparting, through example, that we

- value being lifelong learners committed to the self-appraisal of our own continuing competence;
- foster partnerships between academia and practice;
- effectively communicate the value of occupation in promoting the lifelong health and well-being of persons;
- provide leadership and advocacy to create a person-centered, proactive health care system;
- actively participate in the occupational therapy professional community;
- validate occupational therapy services through outcome research;
- practice in an ethical and competent framework that supports best practice;
- create practice opportunities;
- embrace innovation; and
- creatively manage through change.

The American Occupational Therapy Association affirms its commitment to education through the launching of this publication. I believe *Innovations in Occupational Therapy Education* will be an important resource to reach our goal—to prepare future occupational therapy practitioners to successfully meet the challenges of the future. Congratulations to the Editor and Editorial Board on this inaugural edition.

Karen Jacobs, EdD, OTR/L, CPE, FAOTA, is President, American Occupational Therapy Association, Inc., and Clinical Associate Professor, Department of Occupational Therapy, Boston University, Boston, Massachusetts.

Toward Educational Excellence

Cynthia Hughes Harris

Since the beginning of time, attempts have been made to understand education in terms of the process of teaching and its anticipated results—that of learning. Thus, it is no surprise that occupational therapy, through the American Occupational Therapy Association's Commission on Education, as well as other organizational bodies, continues to strive for excellence in its educational undertakings. It is fitting and timely that the publication *Innovations in Occupational Therapy Education* (IOTE) emerges as yet another forum for educational issues to be questioned, and perhaps resolved as the profession continues to define itself and its contributions in the 21st century.

To discuss education allows a return to Socrates, who attempted to organize and systematize the intellectual abilities. He suggested that "knowledge is virtue and ignorance is evil" (Socrates, 4th century B.C.). For Socrates, education was necessary for a meaningful moral life. Later, John Dewey (1916) viewed education as the "reconstruction or reorganization of experience which…increases the ability to direct the course of subsequent experience" (p. 10). And, it was Whitehead (1929) who argued that education is the "acquisition of the art of utilization of knowledge" (p. 23).

If occupational therapy responds to such monumental descriptions of education, the role of teacher, the actual educator, assumes a position of monumental importance. IOTE is an ideal opportunity to explore the prototype of teacher for the practice of occupational therapy as it is envisioned for today and into tomorrow. What kind of teacher can respond to the educational demands that confront the profession while rising to the challenges of the esteemed educators of history? In this way of thinking, the occupational therapy educator must be one who challenges the "taken-for-granted," problem solves solutions, and questions perceived realities. A teacher of this type engages in such exercises not only for students, but also for self. These teachers are philosophers, scientists, artists, citizens, and perhaps even activists, but only if they remain open to the neverending possibilities of the field. Students approach such teachers for questions, not answers, for possibilities, not prescriptions, because these teachers are both seeker and guide, disciple and mentor.

As we look toward tomorrow, we recognize that the successful occupational therapy educator is able to exemplify similar methods and approaches to those that are expected of students. Three such areas can be used to illustrate such a premise. First, the *art of inquiry* into unique situations is indispensable if teaching is conceived as a complex endeavor requiring continuous awareness, reevaluation, and adjustment. Inquiry becomes an important component of both teaching and learning, which makes it a central concern of education.

A second area of skill for teacher and student is that of *reflection*. Reflective action entails the active, persistent, and careful consideration of any belief as well as routine action that is guided primarily by tradition, external authority, and circumstance. The former describes thoughtful, intentional choice, whereas the latter suggests reactive behavior. The success of occupational therapy educators is dependent on active reflection. In this context, reflection is more than just thinking. For the needs of occupational therapy, reflection is thinking rigorously, critically, and systematically about the practices and problems of importance to the profession.

Critique is a third approach that can be common to both teachers and students. Critique involves the ability for both groups to ask their own questions and seek their own answers. Critique follows practical inquiry and reflection and facilitates the move from insight to decision and from understanding to action.

Increased levels of educational complexity and uncertainty characterize both occupational therapy and society as a whole. Approaches to preparing students for practice are numerous and elaborate. We cannot infuse the above methods, but we can value, practice, and examine them within our commissions, committees, task forces, and publications. If so, occupational therapy education can be a successful leader and a successful follower in the journey of the profession toward excellence.

References

Dewey, J. (1916). *Democracy and education.* New York: Macmillan.

Socrates. (4th century B.C.). *Diogenes laertius: Book II* (section 31; R.D. Hicks, Trans.). Boston: Harvard University Press.

Whitehead, A. N. (1929). *The aims of education and other essays.* New York: Macmillan.

Cynthia Hughes Harris, PhD, OTR, FAOTA, is Chairperson, American Occupational Therapy Association Commission on Education, and Director and Associate Professor, Programs in Occupational Therapy, Columbia University, New York, New York.

Scholarship Revisited: Expanding Horizons and Guidelines for Evaluation of the Scholarship of Teaching

Charlotte Brasic Royeen

In a major work by Glassick, Huber, and Maeroff (1997), the notion of what constitutes scholarship was expanded beyond the traditional realm of discovery of new knowledge (i.e., research) to include three other important domains.

1. The scholarship of teaching
2. The scholarship of integration
3. The scholarship of application

Publication of this debut yearly monograph, *Innovations in Occupational Therapy Education* (IOTE), provides a means for dissemination of writings in occupational therapy on the scholarship of teaching. Thus, the American Occupational Therapy Association is to be commended for sponsoring this journal, and the Editor, Pat Crist, is to be commended for organizing and facilitating the effort.

By providing a focus on the scholarship of teaching, IOTE challenges us to continue to examine what constitutes excellence in this area. I submit that evaluation of the scholarship of teaching should be made on the basis of the evaluation criteria posed by Glassick et al. (1997). They provide six criteria.

1. Are there clear goals?
2. Is adequate preparation reflected?
3. Have appropriate methods been used?
4. Are there notable results from the scholarship?
5. Is the scholarship effectively communicated?
6. Is there an evaluative component?

Each of these will be briefly addressed as applied toward the scholarship of teaching.

Clear goals provide a direction or a focus of scholarly endeavor. When applied to teaching, this does not mean just the delineation of behaviorally based objectives. Rather, clear goals may mean a view toward a grander vision, a plan or pattern of intent and direction. Occupational therapy is challenged to articulate such a grand vision in education. This journal is a beginning, but only a beginning, down that path.

Reflection of adequate preparation requires that we, as educators, do our best to provide the optimal learning experience for a student or client given the context of instruction. Adequate preparation ranges from diligent planning days or weeks before actual instruction to a lifetime of study and reflection in a given area or topic. The standard for adequate preparation for a professional means the ability to extemporaneously speak about a topic for up to a half hour, to answer questions about the topic in a reasonable and knowledgeable manner, and to clearly understand what one does not know about a topic or process. Thus, adequate reflection produces a humble teacher.

Appropriate methods for the scholarship of teaching, and for evaluation of it, are in considerable flux. Teaching itself is changing faster than we can educate ourselves. Technological innovations make the instructional technology of today nearly obsolete by tomorrow. Furthermore, the evaluation of educational instruction is likewise in flux. Innovation in the use of mixed methods that combine quantitative and qualitative research strategies to evaluate learning will likely be the eventual victor in the competition to capture educational experiences in a legitimate, scholarly manner.

Importance of the results of the scholarship of teaching need not be held to the traditional form of comparison with a level of probability of a=0.05. In other words, educational scholarship is not just comparing two groups of students on perfomance by using an experimental or quasiexperimental design. Rather, the old-fashioned notion of common sense criteria can be used, assuming that appropriate logical argumentation accompanies the evaluation of interpretation of the criteria.

Effective communication of the scholarship may be the written word, as is the norm, but I look forward to the day when analysis and content of education is conveyed not just by text but by symbols ranging from mathematical formulations to artistic expression. We need not be limited by the past methods of scholarly communication—we are limited only by our shortcomings and cultural norms.

Finally, but perhaps most important, are the evaluative components of a scholarly work. Does the author, or creator, have a sense of the worth or value of the work? Is the work framed in context and in terms of societal need? Can one see the strengths and areas of weaknesses of the scholarship?

Occupational therapy is moving toward exciting work by introducing this journal dedicated to the scholarship of teaching. I hope that this brief review of innovations in scholarship related to education and evaluation, thereof, provides another piece to move along this journal of learning in which we are all engaged.

Reference

Glassick, C. E., Huber, M. T., & Maeroff, G. I. (1997). *Scholarship assessed: Evaluation of the professoriate* (an Ernest L. Boyer Project of the Carnegie Foundation for the Advancement of Teaching). San Francisco: Jossey-Bass.

Charlotte Brasic Royeen, PhD, OTR, FAOTA, is Chairperson, Education Special Interest Section, American Occupational Therapy Association, and Associate Dean for Research and Professor in Occupational Therapy, School of Pharmacy and Allied Health Professions, Creighton University, Omaha, Nebraska.

With this first edition of *Innovations in Occupational Therapy Education* (IOTE), a vision of many occupational therapy educators, both academic and fieldwork, has finally been materialized. The purpose of this peer-reviewed annual publication will be to disseminate information regarding quality fieldwork and academic educational approaches. The 1995–1998 American Occupational Therapy Association (AOTA) Education Special Interest Section Steering Committee, which included Dr. Janette Schkade, Dr. Aimee Luebben, Professor Annette Port, and myself, created the proposal to establish this publication to provide a conduit for sharing ideas and knowledge to promote "best practices" in occupational therapy education and provide a historical accounting of our educational development. As part of the ongoing effort to enhance the support of our educators, AOTA agreed to publish IOTE as an annual review with a rotating Editorial Board, every member with a 3-year term of office. I was honored to be appointed as the first Editor to bring the publication through its founding year. I thank the Editorial Board for a stellar year of successful work as we laid the foundation for this publication. The initial content for this first annual review is focused, substantive, innovative, and fore-telling of future quality as IOTE becomes more established.

As health care providers, we are aware of major changes affecting occupational therapy education. Therefore, the emergence of IOTE is well timed to facilitate the sharing of innovative educational strategies and scholarship regarding fieldwork and academic practices and management.

In the founding year, several questions frequently arose. Here is a response to those questions.

1. As indicated in IOTE's mission, we are interested in innovative fieldwork and academic teaching and management approaches from all levels of education. Manuscripts must be written in a scholarly manner but do not require research processes. However, some form of outcome data or discussion about potential measurement approaches is highly recommended to demonstrate effectiveness or efficiency of the presented educational innovation.

2. IOTE will be published once a year until the number of quality manuscripts and the number of purchased copies demonstrate support for this review. Subscriptions are not required.

3. The rise of consumer education is recognized by the Editorial Board. This

role is not currently included in IOTE. However, we welcome articles that provide information on this topic due to its intensifying prevalence in service delivery and the acknowledgment that educational approaches used in the classroom, laboratory, or fieldwork are not readily adaptable to this emerging area of practice.

The IOTE Editorial Board represents a wide variety of interests and back-grounds. The Board offered the following list of important topics for future study in occupational therapy education. The list is to stimulate ideas and is not all-inclusive of critical educational approaches warranting study or IOTE consideration.

A Partial List of Current Occupational Therapy Education Questions

General

- What are the similarities and differ-ences between certified occupational therapy assistant and occupational therapist clinical reasoning? What learning methods are best suited to student learning and practice?

- What constitutes good laboratory and fieldwork experiences?

- How are professional identity, self-con-fidence, and skill expertise developed?

- How is ethics education incorporated into the classroom and fieldwork? How is this learning facilitated in the class-room and during fieldwork?

- What do students learn about diversi-ty? How is this information used during performance with peers, clients, and communities?

- What educational strategies promote lifelong learning?

- What is consumer satisfaction with our educational programs from student and public perspectives?

Academic

- What leadership styles promote faculty member development and department growth?

- How can students who are good recall or rote learners of details transition successfully to application, synthesis, and clinical decision making?

- What is our faculty configuration and performance? How does this influence faculty tenure or promotion, the devel-opment of occupational therapy, and the department's value to the campus?

- How does a specific instructional strat-egy promote learning or professional goals?

- What are the comparative outcomes from distance learning, compressed formats, and traditional scheduling?

- Are there different educational out-comes and professional activities of faculty members and graduates on the basis of level of education offered or institutional type?

Fieldwork

- How is theory versus clinical skill com-petence used during fieldwork and for professional practice?

- What is needed to be a successful field-work educator or student?

- How do the various formats for field-work affect professional socialization?

- What enhances or detracts from con-sumer satisfaction with student practi-tioners?

- What is the influence of various types of supervision and fieldwork on stu-dent learning outcomes?

■ What approaches are successful in dealing with the problem student?

In closing, special recognition goes to Karen Nootbaar who assisted greatly in the development of IOTE. She served as assistant to the Editor and provided exemplary presentation of initial materials while facilitating both Editorial Board and author communication. Her organizational efficiency, professional demeanor, and continual accuracy have been greatly appreciated.

I thank the authors and AOTA leaders who submitted their important thoughts and work to the first edition of IOTE. Each provides an innovative contribution to quality academic and fieldwork education in occupational therapy. Most occupational therapy practitioners are educators in their day-to-day jobs and either serve as fieldwork or academic educators. Thus, the work contained in this and future editions is essential information for the practice of these integral occupational therapy roles and related functions.

I invite readers to consider participation in IOTE processes either through submitting manuscripts, serving on the Editorial Board, or providing the Editor with comments or suggestions. Information about these processes is located on the AOTA Web page (www.aota.org). Purchase your own copy and make sure that every occupational therapy library has a copy, too. This and future editions of IOTE will support the role of occupational academic or fieldwork educators and leaders because "Our Practice Is Education!"*

Patricia A. Crist, PhD, OTR/L, FAOTA

Founding Editor, IOTE

Chair and Professor, Duquesne University

*The motto of the 1995–1998 Education Special Interest Section Standing Committee.

Aim & Scope

By focusing on practical application and research in occupational therapy education, *Innovations in Occupational Therapy Education* (IOTE) will facilitate the sharing of contemporary educational approaches among academic and fieldwork educators. By highlighting the best practices in education, the annual, peer-reviewed publication will serve as a resource for educators. Over time, this will become a historical document of the developments in occupational therapy education. Content will include but not be limited to:

- instructional methods;
- fieldwork process, supervision, and models;
- professional development of educators and students;
- administration of academic and fieldwork programs; and
- comparative or applied research in education.

Manuscripts on these topics, broadly construed, are encouraged.

The sponsorship of IOTE by the American Occupational Therapy Association is an affirmation of the association's commitment to advancing the practice of education through scholarship and the communication of viable strategies and resources.

This annual review seeks to publish original manuscripts pertaining to academic and fieldwork education. Manuscripts on a broad range of subjects of potential interest to occupational therapy educa-

tors will be considered. Of particular interest are manuscripts that:

- demonstrate the value and effectiveness of instructional models and methodologies during fieldwork and academic activities;
- describe contemporary learning approaches by using innovative technology, methods, or resources to promote critical thinking, clinical reasoning, and skill acquisition;
- advance the conceptual basis for the practice occupational therapy education;
- propose inventive approaches to instructing students in roles including, but not limited to, scholarship, consultation, case management, management, and leadership, as well as professional socialization to the practitioner role in general;
- provide a forum to discuss approaches to educational management and leadership; and
- support the development of faculty members, fieldwork educators, scholars, and academic leaders.

Additionally, scholarly dialogue is encouraged through Letters to the Editor and invited Commentary. Occasionally, the editor will select discussants to critique accepted manuscripts, and such commentary will be published after the designated articles. Readers are welcome to submit thoughtful letters to the editor pertaining to content published in IOTE. Other features include Briefs, which presents concise summaries of new educational approaches; Reviews, which features amplified summaries of educational approaches; and Commentary, which presents scholarly argument of an education-related view or emerging issue.

Full-length manuscripts are evaluated through a blind review process, and selection is made on the basis of relevance to the profession, scientific merit, timeli-ness, and scholarly excellence. All contributors are required to assign exclusive copyright to the American Occupational Therapy Association, and assurance must be given that manuscripts are not under consideration for publication elsewhere. Potential contributors should consult submission guidelines published in the review under Information for Authors.

.

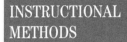

Deus Ex Machina:
Distance Education as Solution?

Susan C. Burwash

Kalya Cotkin

Susan C. Burwash, MSc, OTR, OT(C), is Assistant Professor, and Kalya Cotkin, MS, OTR, is Program Director, Department of Rehabilitation Sciences, Occupational Therapy Program, Texas Tech University Health Sciences Center, Lubbock, Texas.

This article describes an occupational therapy program that uses interactive television to teach entry–level students at three sites. The question of whether there are differences between sites in students grades has been answered; however, student and faculty member concerns about qualitative aspects of distance education have not been answered. One program's experience with distance education is described in the context of pertinent education research, and recommendations are made for addressing the challenges of teaching and learning at a distance.

T HE DICTIONARY DEFINES *DEUS EX MACHINA* AS "A PERSON OR thing…that appears or is introduced suddenly and…provides a contrived solution to an apparently insoluble problem" (*Merriam-Webster's Collegiate Dictionary*, 1993. Is distance education academia's latest *deus ex machina*? What are the costs and benefits of using a distance education approach in occupational therapy education? What should occupational therapy programs considering a move to distance education consider in making their decision?

Although distance education has been around for nearly 150 years, the newest technological advances allow for groundbreaking development (Schlosser & Anderson, 1994). New media allow for sustained two-way communication. Digitalization of print materials allows Internet users access to vast libraries of information. E-mail, live interactive television, the World Wide Web, on-line chat rooms, and database access have all decreased the distance of time and space in distance education (Hawkridge, 1995). Distance education has become an increasingly popular idea as these new technologies become available and as the costs associated with using them decrease.

This article will describe some of the concerns arising from one occupational therapy program's ongoing experience with distance education. A person–environment–occupation framework will be used to review some of the pertinent distance education research, describe some of the options being considered in the ongoing development of this program, and list recommendations for other occupational therapy programs considering the adoption of a distance education approach.

Occupational Therapy Programs and Distance Education

Current Status

Initially, occupational therapy programs have not rushed to adopt new technologies for education of student practitioners (McNurlen, Gilkeson, & Drake, 1996). A recent distance education survey (Angelo & Zukas, 1997) found that only 15%

of occupational therapy education programs were using distance learning in their programs—mostly at the postprofessional level. "Among the 89 programs not presently offering distance learning, 42 (47%) said they were planning or maybe planning to offer distance learning in the future…80% expect to do so in about 2 years" (p. 1). Programs responding to the survey noted reservations about the cost and reliability of equipment, as well as student and faculty issues such as concerns about student isolation, less active learning, diminished contact between students and faculty members, anxiety about using the technology, and students' feelings about the equality of educational experience they receive compared with peers in traditional classroom or laboratory settings.

One Program's Experience

Program description and rationale for distance education approach. Since 1995, the Occupational Therapy Program at Texas Tech University Health Sciences Center (TTUHSC, Lubbock, TX) has used a live interactive television system (which TTUHSC has dubbed *HealthNet*) to teach occupational therapy and physical therapy students at three sites spread 300 miles from north to south. Lectures are delivered to all three campuses by way of interactive television by faculty members at any of the sites with laboratory instruction taking place at each local site. Students interact with local faculty members face to face during lectures and laboratories, and with faculty members from other sites via HealthNet, e-mail, telephone, fax, and faculty member visits to each site. The approach chosen by TTUHSC most clearly resembles the "distributed classroom" model of distance education described by the Institute for Distance Education (University System of Maryland, 1997). In this model, a classroom-based course is extended from one locale to one or more other locales, and faculty members and the institution manage both the instructional schedule and sites.

TTUHSC's educational initiative was designed to make the occupational therapy program accessible to students living in three largely rural areas of west Texas and to increase the overall number of students in the program. The community and state support for this initiative, which brings the program to students living in these areas, results from the assumption that students already living in the areas might be more likely to apply to a program that lets them complete a degree in a locale close to home where they are more likely to remain after graduation. The initiative is also expected to remediate the long-term problem of insufficient numbers of occupational therapy practitioners in these areas.

TTUHSC program outcomes. TTUHSC research to date has focused primarily on student grades as outcome measures, and, as Schlosser and Anderson (1994) and Russell (n.d.) predicted, the results indicated no major difference in grades between campuses. By using data from 1996 to 1998 and by using analysis of covariance to adjust for entering cumulative grade-point average (GPA), Merrifield & Lanier (1998) found that there were no major differences between student grades at the three separate originating (or different) sites for three first-year courses. In addition, no major differences were found between campuses in first-year cumulative GPAs adjusted by entering cumulative GPAs.

Issues. As the research literature summarized in Schlosser and Anderson (1994) and Russell (n.d.) suggested, TTUHSC students and faculty members had concerns about operational aspects of the distance education component of the program that included quality of video and audio transmission, orientation to the system, ongoing technical support, and equity of resources between sites. Students and faculty members identified (through course evaluations, student–faculty discussions, and faculty reflection) some valued aspects of occupational therapy education that can be called the "spiritual" elements, which may be endangered if not explicitly considered in distance education curriculum design. These include interaction between students and faculty members (the sense of knowing and being known), cohesion between student groups, and opportunities for the informal discussion of professional and academic issues that often occurs between faculty members and students as they encounter each other in hallways and offices. Faculty members commented that some students (and some faculty and guest lecturers) appeared to be intimidated by the cameras and microphones in the classrooms, that some instructors seemed to use the medium to be a "sage on the stage" instead of a coach at the sidelines, and that some students responded to the lack of an instructor in the classroom by engaging in unprofessional behavior such as talking during guest lecturer's presentations, playing with the camera, and purposely distracting their classmates during student presentations. These problems echo some of the concerns about distance education voiced in the survey described earlier.

Analyzing Distance Education From an Occupational Therapy Perspective

Occupational Performance Issues in Distance Education

As distance education approaches become increasingly prevalent, how can occupational therapy educators individualize and personalize a basically impersonal medium? How do we ensure that we know our students well enough to be able to stay student–centered when using a distance education approach? How do we develop distance education programs where the perceived benefits outweigh the perceived costs for both students and faculty members? Some of the answers may lie in analyzing the interaction of persons and environments with the occupations of teaching and learning at a distance. The distance education literature has some possible answers to these questions.

Person-Related Factors

When personal characteristics are viewed as part of the equation, programs considering adopting a distance education approach may want to review student selection criteria, faculty member recruitment, and current faculty skills with an eye to the distance education literature. Distance education research has tended to focus mostly on student variables and media comparisons.

Student Recruitment Considerations

Although the research is not conclusive, if success in distance education is defined as course completion, then students who enter programs with higher grades, who have an expectation of earning a degree while maintaining their high academic standards, who have an internal locus of control, and who prefer people-oriented to object-oriented content are more likely to be successful (Coggins, 1988; Dille & Mezak, 1991). Other distance education research has indicated the importance of student skills in active listening and ability to work independently (Charp, 1994). Given these findings and given that occupational therapy programs tend to recruit and admit students who have high grades and expectations of continuing academic success, who have a specific degree in mind when entering the program, and who have an interest in working with people rather than objects, perhaps the distinguishing factors to evaluate when selecting students for a program with a distance education focus would be students with an internal versus external locus of control, active listening skills, and an ability to work independently. The media used by the distance education program, student computer literacy, and what Shapiro and Hughes (1996) called *information literacy* may be important to evaluate before admission and to foster within the curriculum so that students can use the course media with skill and competently access and evaluate on-line information sources.

The student selection process for the TTUHSC occupational therapy program does not include an evaluation of all of these factors, although faculty members are currently investigating various tools that might be helpful in evaluating applicants. The challenge, as always, is to find tools that are quick, easy to use, valid, and reliable.

Faculty Member Skills and Attitudes

Program directors must identify critical characteristics of faculty members involved in the design and delivery of distance education. Interestingly, there has been little distance education research that examines this variable. The assumption appears to be that good teachers will be good teachers regardless of the media used; however, mastery of distance education approaches requires a wide array of skills, some of which may be new to faculty members more accustomed to face-to-face teaching methods. Distance education approaches tend to require well-developed teamwork skills. Boettcher (1998) described the "unbundling" of courses that frequently occurs with distance education—a team becomes responsible for developing and delivering courses, where before, all of those tasks were the faculty member's responsibility. This approach suggests that, in addition to being content experts, faculty members need to be skilled team players who are aware of technology if not adept in using every aspect of it. They must be organized, willing, and able to prepare their materials well in advance of the course and able to work with the team to create an interactive educational experience where "simply accessing information is not enough… information must be shared, critically analyzed, and applied in order to become knowledge" (Garrison, 1990, p. 13). Schlosser and Anderson (1994) described the new skills educators must learn as they become involved in distance education:

> … understanding the nature and philosophy of distance education; identifying learner characteristics at distant sites; designing and developing interactive courseware to suit new technology; adapting teaching strategies to deliver instruction at a distance; organizing instructional resources in a format suitable for independent study; training and practice in the use of telecommunications systems; becoming involved in organization, collaborative planning, and decision-making; evaluating student achievement, attitudes, and perceptions at distant sites; dealing with copyright issues. (pp. 32–37)

All of this learning takes time, training, and support. Sherry (1996) noted that Apple Classrooms of Tomorrow (ACOT) research in kindergarten through grade 12 suggested that most teachers using new media and environments progress through a 3-stage sequence of survival, mastery, and effect. Sherry further noted that it may take teachers 2 or more years to

> …change their focus from being anxious about themselves, their new physical environment, equipment malfunctions, and student misbehavior to anticipating problems and developing alternative strategies, exploring software more aggressively, sharing ideas more freely, increasing student motivation and interest, and using technology to their advantage. (p. 12)

This transition period can be initially daunting for faculty members. New faculty members who now have one more set of learning tasks to master, faculty members who have been successful in other teaching environments and do not see a need for change, and faculty members who are not comfortable with technology may have initial difficulty embracing a distance education program. Most programs do not have the option of recruiting faculty members who are already skilled in distance education methods. As a recent survey (American Occupational Therapy Association, 1998) showed, there is a chronic shortage of occupational therapy faculty members; programs are likely to have difficulty finding faculty members who are technologically adept in addition to being content experts, competent researchers, and creative teachers.

TTUHSC has struggled with faculty recruitment. This may be, in part, related to the geographic location of the program, but it reflects the concerns that potential faculty members have about their skills in using a distance education approach and about the challenges of using distance education technology when building the highly valued interactive learning environments in which many faculty members have previously worked and studied. Members of the clinical community have been somewhat apprehensive about teaching with technology, and this has made it somewhat more difficult to recruit clinicians as guest lecturers.

Facilitators and Other Support Staff Members

The distributed classroom model of distance education relies heavily on the contribution of the site facilitator. The role of the facilitator varies; in general, his or her role is to assist students in remote classrooms, problem solve equipment malfunctions in conjunction with the technical staff members, supervise examination and quiz sessions, and assist the off-site instructor. ACOT (1992) research identified several common skills needed by successful facilitators.

■ Address student behavior and attitudes

■ Manage the classroom environment

■ Address technical issues

■ Understand and work with classroom dynamics

Some programs, including the physical therapy program at TTUHSC, use credentialed teachers or other faculty members as site facilitators. Because of faculty shortages, the occupational therapy program at TTUHSC does not currently do this, and instead has hired facilitators from the community with various backgrounds. In general, the problems with such an arrangement are that facilitators do not view themselves as integral members of the teaching team, and students do not always recognize the authority vested in the facilitator.

The contributions of other staff members are crucial to the success of a distance education course or program. Responsive technical support staff members, whether on site or at a distance, and clerical staff members who coordinate communication between sites and ensure that print and other materials are available to students and faculty members are essential. Faculty member access to staff members with expertise in instructional design can be important for faculty members just beginning to teach a distance education course or program.

At TTUHSC, each site has an administrative secretary and a HealthNet technical support person. The HealthNet system has an instructional design specialist who orients faculty members to the classroom technology and consults with staff members. Both the technical staff members and the instructional design specialist have been especially helpful in providing technical and moral support for faculty members using the system for the first time. Support is often informal in nature; faculty members consult with each other on developing teaching materials and approaches.

Environmental Factors

When examining environmental variables related to distance education in occupational therapy, physical elements such as equipment, teaching resources, physical space, and the social and cultural environments in which the program is operating must be examined.

Physical

Distance education programs vary widely in the media they use and the type and amount of learning resources they provide to students. Providing various resources appears to increase student satisfaction (Schlosser & Anderson, 1994). Picking a combination of media that encourages interactivity is important. A study by Bauer and Rezabek (1992) showed that students are more likely to verbally participate in audioconferencing than videoconferencing and are most likely to participate in a traditional classroom. At TTUHSC, use of various media and modalities (i.e., interactive television, video, hands-on laboratory activities, seminars, student presentations, poster sessions) and an approach that combines distance and on-site teaching is used to encourage student participation.

Most distance education programs provide learning materials and access to library resources, but many do not need or attempt to provide a dedicated physical environment. Given the nature of occupational therapy professional education, it is difficult to imagine how a distance education program could offer all of the required elements without some centralized laboratory space and resources for students.

The TTUHSC program provides dedicated laboratory space at two campuses; at the third, students use the resources of a local health care facility for their laboratory sessions. All campuses have a medical library, although access to resources is somewhat easier at the central campus. This inequity is commented on by students, as are perceived inequities in computer access, and may skew students' cost–benefit calculation when analyzing their experience with this program.

Social

Lave and Wenger (1991) described learning in professions and disciplines as taking place primarily within communities of practice. The newcomer moves from the periphery to the center of the community through interactions with members of the community that provide learning experiences for the neophyte. Occupational therapy students move into their community of practice through interactions in the classroom, laboratory, and clinical setting. Distance education programs must pay particular attention to the social environments they create to ensure that there are many opportunities for interaction and for participation in the work of the community of practice. Sherry (1996) noted that interactivity goes beyond audio and video media and includes the connections students make with the distant faculty members, local faculty and staff members, and their colleagues.

The occupational therapy program at TTUHSC attempts to build a community of practice for students in several ways. Students spend their first semester together at the main campus where they all take an anatomy class together and have opportunities to meet and work with their student colleagues. Faculty members at the main campus have an opportunity to meet students in informal social settings during the summer. During fall and winter semesters, faculty members are expected to visit and teach from each of the regional campuses at least once per semester. Students are introduced to their regional community of practice through interaction with the clinicians who teach some of the laboratory sections and through the experiences they have in local Level I fieldwork placements.

Cultural

The cultural values of the academic environment influence distance teaching and learning. Faculty members are influenced by the attitudes and policy of university administration. Does administration truly value teaching? Is the development of an effective on-line course or program seen as legitimate scholarly work, or does the institution limit its definition of scholarship to research? Are administrators aware of and willing to support the considerable development time involved in designing a distance education approach? How will getting involved in developing a new course or new approach affect tenure and promotion? Most faculty members will need answers to these questions before they can commit to developing new approaches.

Reflection on Practice and Future Plans

Given the issues identified by faculty members and students and the research findings, what changes might a distance education program such as the one at TTUHSC make? Currently, we are

- considering ways in which we can deliver lecture content in an asynchronous rather than synchronous manner by minimizing the amount of time students spend sitting in centralized classrooms for lectures while retaining laboratory sessions and promoting interaction between faculty members and students through face-to-face interactions and use of electronic media. For example, we plan to redistribute instructor contact time in a clinical reasoning course by replacing the HealthNet lectures with a web site that will have a course syllabus, course content, assignments, student evaluation, and presentation capabilities. We hope to increase interaction and contact by using HealthNet for small, structured seminars for the students at each site, and have the course instructor travel to all sites to conduct laboratory sessions;

▪ reading and discussing the distance education literature and sharing questions and answers with other faculty members;

▪ looking for evaluation methods to assist us in selecting students who will be successful in a distance education program;

▪ discussing ways of enhancing student and faculty computer and information literacy;

▪ looking closely at the skills needed by on-site facilitators, their roles, and the relationship between instructor and facilitator;

▪ addressing resource equity issues;

▪ using quantitative measures to continue to monitor student outcomes, but adding qualitative measures to future studies of process and outcomes (in particular, exploring the social dimensions of the program); and

▪ implementing a revised set of faculty evaluation criteria that takes into consideration the specific demands of teaching at a distance.

Making Distance Education Work: Recommendations

Although the occupational therapy program at TTUHSC is far from having all the answers about what makes an entry-level program work when using a distance education approach, the following suggestions may be helpful to other programs considering distance education approaches.

1. Ensure that you have support from both administration and faculty members; finding distance education "champions" at both levels of the university hierarchy will make your task much easier.

2. Provide training and ongoing support for faculty members, facilitators, and clinical instructors as they move from survival to mastery in using new teaching approaches.

3. Be aware of the development time required to design or transform a course and find ways to ensure that faculty members get that time.

4. Solve technical problems early and ensure that good technical support services are in place.

5. Involve students and the clinical community in planning and evaluating new course methods.

6. Encourage faculty members to experience a distance education course as a learner—being a distance learner provides a new perspective on distance education.

7. Play with the technology—find out what it can do for you and get comfortable with the tools.

8. Pay attention to the social environment that you create for students and faculty members.

9. Address issues of faculty recognition for developing innovative teaching approaches.

10. Most of all, be patient with yourself and your students as you both learn new ways of teaching and learning.

The potential of distance education approaches in occupational therapy education is substantial; for occupational therapy education to realize this potential, we must consider the ways in which we can enhance student and faculty member satisfaction by increasing the benefit of distance education while minimizing the costs. In doing so, distance education becomes less *deus ex machina* and more an enticing option that educators can call on when making decisions about how to teach and one that students can choose when deciding how they learn best. ◼

Acknowledgment

The authors thank H. Merrifield and R. Lanier for sharing their unpublished research data.

References

American Occupational Therapy Association. (1998, July 9). Results of the post-professional education survey. *OT Week, 12,* 15.

Angelo, J., & Zukas, R. (1997, April). *Reaching beyond the classroom: New methods of teaching at the professional level.* Paper presented at the annual conference of the American Occupational Therapy Association, Orlando, FL.

Apple Classrooms of Tomorrow. (1992). *Classroom management: Teaching in high-tech environments: First-fourth year findings* (Classroom Management Research Summary No. 10). Cupertino, CA: Apple Computer.

Bauer, J. W., & Rezabek, L. L. (1992). *The effects of two-way visual contact on student verbal interactions during teleconferenced instruction* (ERIC Document Reproduction Service No. ED 347 972). Springfield, VA: DynEDRS, Inc.

Boettcher, J. V. (1998). How much does it cost to develop a distance learning course? It all depends. *Syllabus, 11,* 56–58.

Charp, S. (1994, April). *Viewpoint: The On-Line Chronicle of Distance Education and Communication, 7*(2) [On-line]. Available: Usenet Newsgroup alt.education. distance.

Coggins, C. C. (1988). Preferred learning styles and their impact on completion of external degree programs. *American Journal of Distance Education, 2,* 25–37.

Dille, B., & Mezak, M. (1991). Identifying predictors of high risk among community college telecourse students. *American Journal of Distance Education, 5,* 24–35.

Garrison, D. R. (1990). An analysis and evaluation of audio conferencing to facilitate education at a distance. *American Journal of Distance Education, 4,* 13–24.

Hawkridge, D. (1995). The big bang theory in distance education. In F. Lockwood (Ed.), *Open and distance learning today* (pp. 3–11). New York: Routledge.

Lave, J., & Wenger, E. (1991). *Situated learning: Legitimate peripheral participation.* Cambridge, England, United Kingdom: Cambridge University Press.

McNurlen, G., Gilkeson, G. E., & Drake, C. S. (1996). Computer-assisted instruction in occupational therapy education. *American Journal of Occupational Therapy, 26,* 890–893.

Merriam-Webster's collegiate dictionary (10th ed.). (1993). Springfield, MA: Merriam-Webster.

Merrifield, H. H., & Lanier, R. (1998, February). *Distance education outcomes in occupational therapy.* Poster session presented at the annual conference and winter meeting of the Association of Schools of Allied Health Professions, Daytona, FL.

Russell, T. L. (n.d.). The no significant difference phenomenon: Part 3: '78–'96 [On-line]. Available: http://tenb.mta.ca/phenom/phenom3.html

Schlosser, C. A., & Anderson, M. L. (1994). *Distance education: Review of the literature.* Washington, DC: Association for Educational Communications and Technology.

Shapiro, J. J., & Hughes, S. K. (1996). Information literacy as a liberal art [On-line]. *Educom review, 31*(2). Available: http://www.educause.edu/pub/er/ review/ reviewarticles/31231.html

Sherry, L. (1996). Issues in distance learning. *International Journal of Distance Education, 1*(4), 337–365 [On-line]. Available: http://www.cudenver.edu/public/ education/sherry/pubs//issues.html

University System of Maryland. (1997). *Three models of distance education* [On-line]. Available: http://www.umuc.edu/ide/modldata.html

Preliminary Study of Learning Through Discussion in Occupational Therapy Education

Charlotte Brasic Royeen

Andrea M. Zardetto-Smith

Maureen E. M. Duncan

Charlotte Brasic Royeen, PhD, OTR, FAOTA, is Chairperson, Education Special Interest Section, American Occupational Therapy Association, Associate Dean for Research and Professor in Occupational Therapy, School of Pharmacy and Allied Health Professions, Creighton University, Omaha, Nebraska.

Andrea M. Zardetto-Smith, PhD, is Assistant Professor, Physical Therapy, School of Pharmacy and Allied Health Professions, Creighton University, Omaha, Nebraska.

Maureen E. M. Duncan, OTD, is Instructor, Occupational Therapy, School of Pharmacy and Allied Health Professions, Creighton University, Omaha, Nebraska.

*Teaching neuroscience in occupational therapy typically involves a tradi-
tional lecture and laboratory instructional format. Yet research suggests
that alternative instructional strategies may better assist students to integrate concepts, master terminology, and increase recall. Thus, pilot investigation of an instructional strategy on the basis of W. F. Hill's Learning
Through Discussion (LTD) was implemented into neuroscience courses by
using first-year occupational therapy doctoral (OTD) students serving as
discussion group leaders with first-year bachelor's degree (BSOT) students
in occupational therapy. The OTD students were oriented to LTD during
their advanced neuroscience class, and the BSOT students were oriented to
the LTD process during a brief class overview in their neuroscience class.
Subsequently, on two separate occasions, the BSOT students were assigned
to discussion groups of 6 to 10 students by using systematic, random
assignment. BSOT students were given the case and guiding questions 2
weeks before the scheduled discussion period. The BSOT students met with
the OTD group leader for 1-hr sessions. Reactions of BSOT (n = 38) and
OTD students (n = 8) were separately evaluated at the completion of the
pilot study. By using a Likert-type scale format that covered questions
ranging from content learned to reported satisfaction with the experience,
both groups responded positively and recommended inclusion of this
instructional method into the traditional instructional curriculum. On the
basis of this pilot study, specific curricular recommendations are made
and delimitations put forth.*

T O BETTER MEET SOCIETAL NEEDS, THE PEW COMMISSION
report, *Health Professions Education for the Future: Schools in
Services to the Nation* (O'Neil, 1993), identified that health care professionals must be educated in the following key areas: communication,
teamwork, cultural sensitivity, problem solving, and ability to learn new information. Although the profession of occupational therapy attempts to meet educational challenges through the *Standards for an Accredited Educational
Program for the Occupational Therapist and the Occupational Therapy
Assistant* (American Occupational Therapy Association [AOTA], 1997), these
standards address *content* of occupational therapy instruction for entry-level
education and do not address *method* of instruction. Analysis of the key areas
identified by the Pew Commission reveals that competence may be best
addressed not only by content of instruction but also by method or instructional
strategy. Thus, instructional strategy is the focus of this article.

Instructional strategy, or how to teach, is at the core of what we do both as occupational therapy practitioners and as academic instructors. However, in occupational therapy we have a dearth of attention paid to the process of education. Consideration of research on education as a process is scant. Review of the *American Journal of Occupational Therapy* and *Occupational Therapy Journal of Research* from 1980 to 1996 revealed that only 18 articles focused on education. And, of those, half concerned fieldwork (Cohn & Frum, 1988; Hamlin, MacRae, & DeBrakeleer, 1995; Kautzmann, 1990) and not instructional methodologies, even though *fieldwork* was not a key term used in the literature search. The lack of published educational research in occupational therapy demonstrates the need for the current series of annual reviews (*Innovations in Occupational Therapy Education*) and the need to evaluate instructional methods for use in occupational therapy.

This article focuses on an instructional strategy called Learning Through Discussion (LTD; Rabow, Charness, Kipperman, & Radcliffe-Vasile, 1994) that provides an innovative instructional method to the more common method of education (i.e., classroom lecture). LTD is a specifically prescribed eight-step directed process of group discussion. These eight steps consist of

1. checking in,
2. defining vocabulary words from an assigned reading,
3. identifying key concepts from the assigned reading,
4. discussing key concepts,
5. applying key concepts to other materials and work,
6. exploring how material applies to discussion group members,
7. evaluating the assigned reading, and
8. evaluating the group (Rabow et al., 1994).

The previously cited Pew Commission report (O'Neil, 1993) skills needed by health care practitioners in the future cannot be developed by using traditional lecture methods of instruction. LTD may be one strategy to promote development of these needed skills. Thus, the focus of this study is an exploration into the use of LTD in an occupational therapy curriculum at Creighton University (Omaha, NE). A preliminary report of this data has previously been published (Royeen & Zardetto-Smith, 1997).

Review of the Literature on LTD

The LTD method of instruction was first introduced as an instructional method by William Fawcett Hill nearly 30 years ago (Rabow et al., 1994). LTD uses an active approach to learning in which students engage in an interactive discussion group. The LTD method has been applied as an instructional method in various educational settings for the past 20 years (Aamodt, 1983; Hall, 1995; Livingston & Gentile, 1995; Zimmer, Wilson, & Bruning, 1974). In almost all cases, the use of case study and group discussion has been found to be an effective means of instruction.

Research examining the LTD approach to education in medical curricula development and implementation has found this instructional method to be an effective educational strategy (Gelula, 1997; Grant, 1993; Herbert, 1993). A recent medical education study (Gelula, 1997) found that medical students who participate in interactive group discussion are able to retain what they learn for longer periods of time than students who engage in traditional classes with a lecture format. Gelula (1997) stated that, in addition to facilitating active participation, students engaging in discussion groups are better able to integrate previously acquired knowledge with new materials and apply it to clinical settings.

Although numerous studies have found that participation in discussion groups is a highly effective instructional methodology (Katz, 1990; Royeen, 1995), little has been written regarding the integration of discussion groups with the LTD instructional method in occupational therapy instructional curricula (Toth-Cohen, 1995; Tyressenaar, 1993). Recently, there has been a renewed interest in occupational therapy instruction and the use of problem-based learning (PBL), which incorporates principles of LTD (Katz, 1990; Royeen, 1995; VanLeit, 1995; Watson & West, 1996). Cahill and Madigan (1984) described the importance of incorporating alternative learning methods into occupational therapy curricula. Further, Katz (1990) and Raveh (1995) emphasized the importance of matching instructional method to student learning style.

Although it is generally recognized that educational methods are an important part of curriculum design and implementation, little research has been devoted to this topic. Additional investigation into the effectiveness of using LTD methods as an instructional strategy in occupational therapy student education is warranted.

Methods

Participants

Participants in this investigation were two cohorts of occupational therapy students. One cohort consisted of junior-level undergraduate students enrolled in the second semester of occupational therapy baccalaureate education who were taking a required course in neuroanatomy (BSOT students). The second cohort consisted of students enrolled in an advanced neuroscience course given in the second semester of an occupational therapy doctorate postprofessional course of study (OTD students). In these two cohorts, some students were absent during the educational intervention due to illness and scheduling conflicts. Thus, cohort 1 (BSOT students) consisted of 38 participants (out of a potential 50), and cohort 2 (OTD students) consisted of 8 participants (out of a potential 12). The course director for the neuroanatomy course was a doctorate-level, non–occupational therapy practitioner and neuroscientist. The course director for the OTD advanced neuroscience course was a doctorate-level occupational therapy practitioner. Because this was a preliminary study using two case scenarios, content validation and reliability of the questionnaire were not calculated.

Procedure

During the spring semester of 1997, the OTD students were oriented to the process of LTD in their course. They read the book *William Fawcett Hill's Learning Through Discussion* (Rabow et al., 1994) and discussed aspects of it during a class session. These OTD students then served as the group leaders for the discussions to be convened with the BSOT students. Serving as a group leader was a requirement for the class.

Students enrolled in the BSOT program were taking a BSOT neuroscience class. Two discussion sessions of cases were planned in their course. The lead author oriented the BSOT students to the LTD process with a brief overview in the BSOT neuroscience course. On two separate occasions, the BSOT students were assigned to discussion groups by using systematic, random assignment. BSOT students were provided the individual case for consideration 2 weeks before the discussion period. Thus, the case discussions occurred in conjunction with traditional lecture presentation of neuroscience information and were scheduled to occur approximately halfway through the semester. The cases were selected to highlight and refine main neuroscience concepts from an occupational therapy clinical point of reference.

Approximately 9 to 10 BSOT students met with their assigned discussion group leader (an OTD student) for approximately 1.5 hr for each session. The students had a different leader each time.

Cases

The case scenarios were selected from previous course materials developed by the lead author for a neuroscience class that used aspects of PBL at Shenandoah University (Winchester, VA). Two cases were selected on the basis of demonstrating fundamental neuroscience principles taught in the BSOT neuroscience course and the prevalence of the underlying neuropathology in occupational therapy practice. One case concerned a person who had a stroke, and the other involved a child with mental retardation and developmental disability. These cases are provided in Appendix A and are modified from materials provided by the American Occupational Therapy Foundation (AOTF) and AOTA.

Evaluation

BSOT and OTD students were asked to evaluate their LTD experiences 1 week after completion of the second discussion groups. Appendix B presents the evaluation forms used. One form was used by the discussion group leaders, and the other form was used by the students who participated in the discussion.

Results

Table 1 presents the quantitative data of discussion leader evaluation (OTD students) of LTD. The frequency distribution of the modes of the scores presented in Table 1 reveals that, overall, the experience was viewed positively by the discussion group leaders.

Written comments were not grouped thematically due to the small number of study participants and the exploratory nature of the study. Illustrative quotes given in response to each of the nonquantitatively based questions on the questionnaire follow. Selected written comments from question 7, "What do you see as the major benefits of this strategy?" follow.

▪ "Group processing of information. Information is not regurgitated back and allows for different views, questions, and estimates of knowledge."

Table 1
Data Sheet: Tutor Group Leaders Evaluation of Learning Through Discussion

	Ratings		
	3	4	5
Rate the experience you had as a tutor group leader in terms of its adding to your knowledge in neuroscience.	—	5	3
Rate the experience you had as a tutor group leader in terms of learning how to educate occupational therapy practitioners	—	4	4
Rate the experience you had as a tutor group leader in terms of learning about group processes.	1	5	2
Think about other educational experiences you have had in the OTD program. Rate this experience of serving as a tutor to your other educational experiences.	—	5	3
How beneficial do you think it would be to expand the pilot LTD into more of the curriculum?	1	3	4
If you were designing an educational event, would you use LTD strategies?	1	3	4

Note. N = 8. Rating 3 = no beliefs pro or con, Rating 4 = probably likely or probably helpful, Rating 5 = extremely likely or extremely helpful, LTD = learning through discussion, OTD = occupational therapy doctoral.

- "Fosters creative problem solving and assertiveness."

- "Once students overcame their uncomfortableness—it would be a wonderful way to increase communication abilities as well as self-confidence."

- "It was a wonderful learning experience—I learned a great deal about students as learners and how preparedness drives discussion. It required me to reflect on causes—good refreshers. Good learning for students in discussion skills."

- "Iterative. Increases retention. Increases understanding. Great style of learning. Learning confidence of being able to stand before a group as well as to plan and execute the content matter."

- "Made aware of own deficits/areas uncomfortable. Provided opportunity for synthesis and application of information."

- "Builds listening skills. Discussion skills into curriculum versus a separate class. Increases and supports risk taking as a learning strategy."

Selected written comments from question 8, "What do you see as the major problems of this learning strategy?" follow.

- "Doesn't work well with students who are aren't prepared."

- "Need to be in the small group—it isn't lecture teaching."

- "Being comfortable with the process."

- "The lack of preparedness of students. Too large of a group on one of the days. A few terms were not clarified for facilitators."

- "Not effective for some individuals. Shy individuals not as participatory as outspoken individuals."

- "Hard not to lecture during 'dead' or nonspeaking time. Difficult when members had not read the material."

- "Participants and instructor come from a lifetime of learning techniques; it will take time to process and learn."

Selected written comments from question 9, "Do you have any other questions you wish to share?" follow.

- "Fantastic experience, would be great if we could keep same group members and meet one to two times monthly. Great method for preparing us to someday teach!"

- "Great."

- "I really enjoyed the process."

- "This has been a beneficial experience."

- "Some of us were uncertain as to what information was desired due to some of the terminology. It would have been helpful to have an opportunity to overview the case studies and questions prior to class facilitation."

■ "I think it would be a valid learning project to use the OTD students who express interest in education as well as others throughout the curriculum."

Table 2 presents the modes of frequencies of responses from the BSOT student evaluations of the experience. Again, the frequency distribution of the modes of scores presented in Table 2 reveals a positive response to LTD on part of the BSOT students involved.

Selected written comments from the BSOT students follow.

1. "The facilitators were wonderful….Thanks!"
2. "At first the leader taught instead of discussed, which was not so beneficial to the group discussion."
3. "The discussion group leader did a great job."
4. "The discussion group leader was nice and easy to talk with."

Delimitations

The participants of this investigation were a convenience sample, and, thus, generalizability of the findings to all populations of occupational therapy students is not warranted. Careful replication of the current study with concomitant systematic evaluation is required to build on the body of evidence that

Table 2
Data Sheet: Student Evaluation of Learning Through Discussion

	SD	D	U	A	SA
I learned the information.	—	—	—	20	18
I liked this learning activity.	—	—	1	20	17
Compared with lecture format, I learned the information better.	—	1	5	14	18
Compared with other learning activities, I will remember what I learned from this better.	—	1	6	15	16
The learning activity made me uncomfortable.	17	18	2	1	—
Learning in a group is beneficial.	—	—	—	23	15
I had to prepare differently for this than for other classes.	1	9	8	19	1
I would like to repeat this type of learning experience.	—	—	1	17	20

Note. N = 38. SD = strongly disagree, D = disagree, U = undecided, A = agree, SA = strongly agree.

suggests that LTD is an effective instructional strategy for occupational therapy education. The effects of case instruction versus the interaction effect of entry level with clinically experienced occupational therapy practitioners may be examined separately.

Analysis and Discussion

On the basis of the foregoing qualitative and quantitative results, both the cohort of BSOT students and the OTD students viewed the LTD experience in an extremely positive manner. Analysis of the BSOT results in Table 2 shows that 100% of the students either agreed or strongly agreed that they had learned information from the experience. Only 1 student out of 37 found the experience uncomfortable. Of the OTD students, 8 of 8 students agreed that the experience was helpful or extremely helpful in adding to their knowledge of neuroscience. Seven out of the 8 would use the same method as an educational strategy, and 8 out of 8 found it to be an extremely helpful method of educating occupational therapy practitioners. A follow-up probe with BSOT students at the end of the semester revealed the strong, positive view of LTD to be sustained.

Although results from a specific educational study pertain to the curriculum in which the study occurred, the implications thereof may be broader and apply across educational curricula (Neistadt, 1987). What formed the basis for the overwhelming enthusiasm of both the BSOT and OTD students for the experience? The clearly positive results of the study indicate that the results obtained were probably not due to a *Hawthorne effect* (i.e., that by virtue of studying something, it changes its very nature, and a positive response is elicited). This concern could easily be addressed in a future, more complete study that includes a control group.

The results were more likely due to the power of case scenarios in an LTD format or the effect of providing interaction between experienced clinicians (OTD students) with the entry-level (BSOT) students. Creighton University is unique in its occupational therapy curriculum due to the presence of both an entry-level BSOT program as well as a postprofessional program for registered practitioners. With the advent of multilevel educational programs combining entry-level degree students with experienced practitioners seeking advanced degrees, the opportunity to integrate innovative educational methods (i.e., those described in this study) into the curriculum can be further explored.

Summary

This study provided support for the premise that, at the educational levels of baccalaureate and clinical doctorate, LTD is perceived to be an extremely positive learning strategy in both the short and long term. It is recommended that, for programs with multiple levels of students, innovations in education can be implemented by having the more experienced students work with the less experienced students in an LTD format. Continued study into the effects of LTD at all levels of education is warranted. ∎

Appendix A

Cases 1 and 2

Case 1: Cerebrovascular Accident (CVA)

(Courtesy of Pamela M. Dougherty, OTR, and Joetta Zola, OTR)

K. J. was a left-handed man 46 years of age with a family history of cerebral aneurysms. His past medical history included chronic hypertension and a subarachnoid hemorrhage that occurred 10 years ago. K. J. sought medical attention after a bout of severe headaches and visual disturbances. A computerized axial tomography scan indicated a subarachnoid hemorrhage, and an angiography revealed aneurysms on the right anterior, right middle, and left middle cerebral arteries. K. J. had surgery to clip the right anterior aneurysm. Postsurgical recovery was complicated by cerebral vasospasms in the bilateral anterior artery, and hydrocephalus that required placement of a frontal peritoneal shunt 10 days after the aneurysm had been clipped. The patient had numerous medical complications in the 2 weeks before he began rehabilitation.

Guiding Questions

Case: CVA

Date case is presented to students: _____ /_____ /_____

1. What is CVA?
2. What are the relationships among right hemiplegia, left hemiplegia, right CVA, and left CVA?
3. Describe the neural mechanisms involved in a right CVA and a left CVA.
4. What is the circulatory system serving in the spinal cord and brain? Why is it important to a CVA?
5. What are the primary or typical differences between a person with left-sided hemiplegia and right-sided hemiplegia?
6. What is hydrocephalus? Why can it be associated with CVA?

Case 2: Mental Retardation and Developmental Disability

(Courtesy of Nedra Gillette, MA, OTR; this synopsis has been adapted from a narrative prepared during the clinical reasoning studies sponsored by AOTF)

Mark is a boy 11 months of age with glioblastoma who has a partial encephalocele. He has mental retardation involving developmental delay and hydrocephalus, increased tone in his upper extremities, gastroesophogeal reflux, and fluctuating problems related to his chemotherapy treatments. Mark's prognosis from birth has been tenuous. He was born in Germany, the first child for Bob and Martha. He underwent partial surgical resection of the brain tumor in Germany before being transferred to an Army hospital in the states. Confirmation of the brain tumor took more than 2 months. Because of his high morbidity risk, the focus of his medical treatment was on establishing a protocol to eradicate the tumor and control his hydrocephalus. The neurosurgeons placed a ventricular shunt to reduce Mark's hydrocephalus 3 weeks before his discharge. He stayed at the Army hospital for 4 months before his transfer to another state, where the family was reassigned. Occupational therapy was provided 3 to 5 times weekly, as his medical status allowed, during that 4-month period.

Although he appears weak and has low endurance, he can clearly demonstrate his strong will and communicate his feelings. He is visually aware of his surroundings. When he's feeling well, he enjoys sitting up in his stroller or being held by someone in the middle of a crowd of people. He will engage in playful games with reaching and grasping for toys and imitating vocalizations. When he's feeling poorly, he likes to be comforted, cuddled, or just have someone nearby in his field of vision.

He is greatly delayed and exhibits gross motor skills at the 3 to 4-month level, fine motor skills at the 6 to 8-month level, and cognitive functions at the 4 to 5-month level. Mark has never liked being prone, and he becomes irritable with much handling or transitional movements. If his head is kept relatively still, he appears much more comfortable.

Mark's parents are young but appear much older. They are inseparable, always holding hands, staying close to each other, and finishing sentences for each other. The father was deployed to Saudi Arabia until Mark's brain tumor was confirmed, and the Army sent him home on emergency leave. Both parents have maintained a fierce independence and highly guarded privacy from the hospital staff members. It appeared to result from a lack of trust. The parents kept their distance and preferred to let Mark's daily care be handled by staff members. When given opportunities to take him out, they repeatedly refused. At best, they would go for a 2-hr walk, but they would never keep him with them overnight. When the father left to pack up their household goods in Germany, the mother became ill and more withdrawn. She has lost a lot of weight and has been taking tranquilizers. Both of Mark's parents have repeatedly refused supportive counseling.

Guiding Questions

Case: Mental retardation with developmental delay

Date case is presented to students: _____ /_____ /_____

1. What are the neural mechanisms underlying it?
2. What is glioblastoma?
3. What is encephalocele?
4. What is mental retardation?
5. What is developmental delay?
6. What is hydrocephalus?
7. What is increased muscle tone (hypertonicity)?

8. What is a ventricular shunt? How does it work to reduce hydrocephalus?

9. Why does Mark get irritable when prone?

10. Why does Mark get irritable when handled a lot?

11. Why is Mark most comfortable when his head is still?

12. Speculate about what is going on with Mark's parents.

Appendix B

Evaluation of Pilot Learning Through Discussion

Discussion Group Leaders and OTD Students

(Ratings: 1=definitely not likely or definitely not helpful, 2=probably not likely or probably not helpful, 3=no beliefs pro or con, 4=probably likely or probably helpful, 5=extremely likely or extremely helpful)

1. Rate the experience you had as a tutor group leader in terms of its adding to your knowledge in neuroscience.   1   2   3   4   5

2. Rate the experience you had as a tutor group leader in terms of learning how to educate occupational therapy practitioners.   1   2   3   4   5

3. Rate the experience you had as a tutor group leader in terms of learning about group processes.   1   2   3   4   5

4. Think about other educational experiences you have had in the OTD program. Rate this experience of serving as a tutor to your other educational experiences.   1   2   3   4   5

5. How beneficial do you think it would be to expand the pilot LTD into more of the curriculum?   1   2   3   4   5

6. If you were designing an educational event, would you use LTD strategies?   1   2   3   4   5

7. What do you see as the major benefits of this learning strategy?
_____

8. What do you see as the major problems of this learning strategy?
_____

9. Do you have any other comments you want to share?
_____

BSOT Students

Think about the two experiences you have had with LTD. Given these experiences, rate the following.

(Ratings: 1=SD, strongly disagree; 2=D, disagree; 3=U, undecided; 4=A, agree; 5=S, strongly agree)

	SD	D	U	A	SA
1. I learned the information.	1	2	3	4	5
2. I liked this learning activity.	1	2	3	4	5
3. Compared with lecture format, I learned the information better.	1	2	3	4	5
4. Compared with other learning activities, I will remember what I learned from this better.	1	2	3	4	5
5. The learning activity made me uncomfortable.	1	2	3	4	5
6. Learning in a group is beneficial.	1	2	3	4	5
7. I had to prepare differently for this than for other classes.	1	2	3	4	5
8. I would like to repeat this type of learning experience.	1	2	3	4	5

Comments:

_____

_____

_____

References

Aamodt, M. G. (1983). Academic ability and student preference for discussion group activities. *Teaching of Psychology, 10*(2), 117–119.

American Occupational Therapy Association. (1997). Standards for an accredited educational program for the occupational therapist and the occupational therapy assistant [Draft]. *OT Week, 11*(46), A1–A12.

Cahill, R., & Madigan, M. (1984). The influence of curriculum format on learning preference and learning style. *American Journal of Occupational Therapy, 38*, 683–686.

Cohn, E., & Frum, D. (1988). The Issue Is—Fieldwork supervision: More education is warranted. *American Journal of Occupational Therapy, 42*, 325–327.

Gelula, M. H. (1997). Clinical discussion sessions and small groups. *Surgical Neurology, 47*(4), 399–402.

Grant, P. (1993). Formative evaluation of a nursing orientation program: Self-paced vs. lecture-discussion. *Journal of Continuing Education in Nursing, 24*(6), 245–248.

Hall, K. (1995). Learning modes: An investigation of perceptions in five Kent classrooms. *Educational Research, 37*(1), 21–32.

Hamlin, R. B., MacRae, N., & DeBrakeleer, B. (1995). Will the Opacich fieldwork model work? *American Journal of Occupational Therapy, 49*, 165–167.

Herbert, C. J. (1993). Curricular changes and improved performance by high-risk students on the National Boards: Part I. *Journal of the Association of Academic Minor Physicians, 4*(3), 82–88.

Katz, N. (1990). Problem solving and time: Functions of learning style and teaching methods. *Occupational Therapy Journal of Research, 10*(4), 221–236.

Kautzmann, L. (1990). Clinical teaching: Supervisors' attitudes and values. *American Journal of Occupational Therapy, 44*, 838–848.

Livingston, J. A., & Gentile, J. R. (1995). Mastery learning and the decreasing variability hypothesis. *Journal of Educational Research, 90*(2), 67–74.

Neistadt, M. E. (1987). Classroom as clinic: A model for teaching clinical reasoning in occupational therapy education. *American Journal of Occupational Therapy, 41*, 631–637.

O'Neil, E. H. (1993). *Health professions education for the future: Schools in service to the nation.* San Francisco: Pew Health Commission.

Rabow, J., Charness, M. A., Kipperman, J., & Radcliffe-Vasile, S. (1994). *William Fawcett Hill's learning through discussion* (3rd ed.). Thousand Oaks, CA: Sage.

Raveh, M. (1995). Configuration of occupational therapy, professionalism and experiential learning—An integrated introductory course. *Occupational Therapy International, 2*(1), 65–78.

Royeen, C. B. (1995). A problem-based learning curriculum for occupational therapy education. *American Journal of Occupational Therapy, 49*, 338–346.

Royeen, C. B., & Zardetto-Smith, A. M. (1997). *Evaluation of learning through discussion using two neuroscience case studies* [Abstract]. Washington, DC: Society for Neuroscience.

Toth-Cohen, S. (1995). Computer-assisted instruction as a learning resource for applied anatomy and kinesiology in the occupational therapy curriculum. *American Journal of Occupational Therapy, 49*, 821–827.

Tyressenaar, J. (1993). Interactive journals: An educational strategy to promote reflection. *American Journal of Occupational Therapy, 49*, 695–702.

VanLeit, B. (1995). Using the ease method to develop clinical reasoning skills in problem-based learning. *American Journal of Occupational Therapy, 49*, 349–353.

Watson, D. E., & West, D. J. (1996). Using problem-based learning to improve educational outcomes. *Occupational Therapy International, 3*(2), 81–93.

Zimmer, J. W., Wilson, E. D., & Bruning, R. H. (1974). Proctor-led discussion groups: A further look. *Journal of Educational Research, 67*(8), 378–381

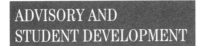

Synergy of Occupational Adaptation and Narrative Metaphor for Student Test Anxiety

Toby Ballou Hamilton

Toby Ballou Hamilton, MPH, OTR/L, is Assistant Professor and Program Director, University of Oklahoma Health Sciences Center, College of Allied Health, Department of Occupational Therapy, Oklahoma City, Oklahoma. A version of this article was presented at the Occupational Adaptation Symposium, March 13–14, 1998, Houston, Texas.

Performance anxiety and its effect on student performance are challenges that perplex occupational therapy academic and clinical educators. Occupational therapy theory, the profession's perspective on the therapeutic use of narrative, and the narrative metaphor combine to form a synergy. This article describes the application of this synergy to reduce a student's test anxiety. The combination of occupational therapy theory and the narrative metaphor suggests ways to apply the intervention for student advisement in the classroom and the clinic.

O CCUPATIONAL THERAPY STUDENTS FACE CHALLENGES IN THE process of learning the knowledge, skills, and attitudes necessary for successful performance as students and beginning practitioners. Many students experience performance anxiety during the didactic and fieldwork segments of their education. Occupational therapy theory can be applied with as much relevance to students as clients. This article describes the synergy of occupational adaptation (OA) theory (Schkade & Schultz, 1992; Schultz & Schkade, 1992), the therapeutic perspective of narrative in the profession, and a narrative metaphor to reduce a student's test anxiety. The combined strengths of the theoretical bases suggest further application for student advisement in the classroom and the clinic.

The OA Frame of Reference

The OA frame of reference describes a normative and internal developmental process by which persons adapt to challenges that arise from interaction with their environments (Schkade & Schultz, 1992; Schultz & Schkade, 1992). Occupational therapy practitioners use OA direct intervention to improve clients' internal adaptation processes to master challenges by enacting adaptive responses that are effective, efficient, and satisfying to themselves and others. Mastery is relative to the particular challenge (Schultz & Schkade, 1992). The internal adaptation process consists of successively generating, enacting, evaluating, and integrating adaptive responses (Schkade & Schultz, 1992). The power of OA lies in its emphasis on the development of internal adaptation to enable persons to meet subsequent challenges with greater success and satisfaction (Schkade & Schultz, 1992; Schultz & Schkade, 1992). The cumulative effect is enhanced internal adaptation in occupational performance.

When faced with a challenge, a person generates a response, acts on it, evaluates how well the response worked for that challenge, and then integrates the response into the adaptive repertoire. Each generation, evaluation, and integration subprocess occurs within three components. Within the generation subprocess, the person selects three components: an energy level that can be primary (focused and intense with high energy expenditure) or secondary (more sophisticated and creative with low energy expenditure); a mode of action that is either existing, modified, or new; and a set of behaviors (repetitive and stuck, random and unfocused, or a mature blend of the other two behaviors). These components are configured into the output of the person's sensorimotor, cognitive, and psychosocial systems to enact the adaptive response. After initiating the adaptive response, the person evaluates and integrates the response for future challenges (Schkade & Schultz, 1992). Educators foster students' internal adaptation processes, as they do for clients, to "narrow the gap between present occupational functioning and the role performance required" (Schultz & Schkade, 1992, p. 920).

The Use of Narrative From the Occupational Therapy Perspective

The use of a person's narrative as a tool for clinical practice and research is familiar to occupational therapy practitioners (Clark, 1993; Clark, Ennevor, & Richardson, 1996; Cohn, 1991; Helfrich & Kielhofner, 1994; Helfrich, Kielhofner, & Mattingly, 1994; Larson & Fanchiang, 1996a, 1996b; Mattingly, 1991; Polkinghorne, 1996). Aspects of narrative that are recognized in occupational therapy include a volitional narrative told from the perspective of the client (Helfrich & Kielhofner, 1994; Helfrich, Kielhofner, & Mattingly, 1994), a story expressing metaphors of volition (Mallinson, Kielhofner, & Mattingly, 1996), a story centered on occupational performance (Clark, 1993; Clark et al., 1996), and a collaborative story about future plans through therapeutic emplotment (Mattingly, 1991). Each of these stories told by clients and practitioners contributes to the therapeutic process.

A person's narrative helps occupational therapy practitioners think about clients (Clark, 1993; Clark et al., 1996; Larson & Fanchiang, 1996b; Mattingly, 1991). It helps both the practitioner and client to understand and give meaning to events (Helfrich & Kielhofner, 1994; Helfrich, Kielhofner, & Mattingly, 1994; Polkinghorne, 1996) and to create or revise the life story (Clark, 1993; Clark et al., 1996; Helfrich & Kielhofner, 1994; Helfrich, Kielhofner, & Mattingly, 1994; Larson & Fanchiang, 1996a; Mallinson, Kielhofner, & Mattingly, 1996; Polkinghorne, 1996). Underlying these applications is the belief that narrative expresses one's life as story and that life is the living out of one's story (Clark, 1993; Clark et al., 1996; Helfrich & Kielhofner, 1994; Helfrich, Kielhofner, & Mattingly, 1994; Polkinghorne, 1996). In occupational therapy, narrative can transform, provide options, inform choices, and envision the future (Clark et al., 1996; Larson & Fanchiang, 1996a; Mattingly, 1991; Polkinghorne, 1996).

The Use of Narrative as Metaphor

In using narrative as metaphor, one's story represents one's life. The plot is the tale of one's agency and details choices made and actions taken. Narrative transformation, or the change in one's story, is a metaphor for the internal adaptation process. The narrative and the internal adaptation process form a reciprocal relationship in which the adaptation process can be stimulated by narrative, and the change in the narrative can indicate the effects of the internal adaptation process. Some of the concepts of use of the narrative metaphor to facilitate OA have been described in occupational therapy (Clark et al., 1996; Polkinghorne, 1996) and in family therapy (Clark et al., 1996; Doan, 1997; Parry & Doan, 1994). Each description assumes the existence of a problem plot that needs revision and outlines a process characterized by nonlinear, simultaneous deconstruction of the problem plot and reconstruction of a revised plot in which agency replaces passivity (Doan, 1997; Parry & Doan, 1994; Polkinghorne, 1996).

Self-stories are interpretations in that people form personal stories from the meanings they give to experience (Bruner, 1990; Polkinghorne, 1996). Practitioners who use the narrative metaphor view unexamined internalized narratives as problematic. Some self-stories can trap the narrator in a plot in which he or she is a victim (Polkinghorne, 1996) of problems that seem impervious to change (Doan, 1997). Because these stories become self-legitimizing (Parry & Doan, 1994) through retelling and living out the story, the problem-saturated plot pushes out all other stories, even those containing contradictory evidence and solutions. The practitioner evokes the problem-saturated plot so that it can be viewed as optional and amenable to change (Parry & Doan, 1994).

Initially, people believe they are controlled by a problem and its effects—often separating the life story into stages before and after the problem (Polkinghorne, 1996). Typically, they view themselves as the problem. Through externalizing and calling the problem "the problem," instead of calling themselves "the problem" (Doan, 1997, p. 5), people free themselves from the constraints (Doan, 1997; Parry & Doan, 1994) that keep them living out the problem plot.

The process of creating the new story, or story revision (Doan, 1997; Parry & Doan, 1994), occurs simultaneously with the deconstruction of the problem plot. The practitioner helps the person look for "unique outcomes" or "lost stories" (Doan, 1997; Parry & Doan, 1994, p. 28) that contradict the problem-saturated story. These form the basis of the revision, which contains a solution (Doan, 1997). The person shapes the revised plot by stating preferences. Working back and forth between the problem plot and the revised plot leads to comparison and clarification of the two plots. By beginning to live out the preferred story through recruiting the support of others (Doan, 1997; Parry &

Doan, 1994), the person transforms the narrative from a victim's plot to an agent's plot (Polkinghorne, 1996).

The Synergy of OA, Narrative, and the Narrative Metaphor

The OA frame of reference, the profession's recognition of the therapeutic nature of narrative, and the narrative metaphor used to facilitate adaptation form a synergy. The synergy advances foundational beliefs in agency, internal change, and enacted adaptation. Accepting the person's narrative and pointing out the possibility of living the preferred plot (Doan, 1997) is consistent with the profession's philosophy of agency (American Occupational Therapy Association, 1979) and a life plot of agency (Polkinghorne, 1996). Each contributes to the belief that people can adapt internally and that, by changing stories, lives can change. The changed narrative is a tale of enacted adaptation.

The approaches offer parallel constructs. The potential for adaptation occurs when adaptation energy, modes, and behaviors no longer achieve results that are effective, efficient, or satisfying; crisis precipitates story revision. The narrative concept that one is stuck in the problem plot and cannot behave otherwise is consistent with the OA construct of being stuck, or hyperstabilized, in primitive behavior and an existing mode.

Not only do the constructs support each other, but also they combine to form a greater strength. By using the narrative metaphor in OA, plot revision and the generation of new adaptive responses are reciprocal processes. The generation of new solutions in narrative form allows vicarious exploration of consequences before the adaptive response is enacted, evaluated, and integrated. The narrative metaphor's unique outcomes or lost stories are simply overlooked, forgotten, adaptive responses that were generated and enacted without adequate evaluation or integration. Contrasting these overlooked responses with the problem plot and personal preferences in story form allows for more thorough engagement of the evaluation and integration subprocesses. Table 1 summarizes these similarities.

Not only can the internal process of OA be initiated by narrative, but also the transformed narrative can identify the process of adaptation. Narrative alone affords self-understanding by telling "a story about one's causes in a new language" (Rorty as cited in Parry & Doan, 1994, p. 17). Through synergy, OA expressed through one's narrative is telling a new story in adaptive language.

Background and the Student's Story

The University Setting as Occupational Environment

The student attended a comprehensive public university that sponsors the state's only professional program and awards a bachelor of science degree in

Table 1
Synergy of OA and the Narrative Metaphor

Constructs	OA	Narrative Metaphor
Evaluation	Articulate the challenge Evaluate the generation, evaluation, and integration subprocesses and products of each	Evoke the problem plot and identify the real problem
Problem	Inability to generate new adaptive responses	Inability to generate a new plot or change an existing one
Nature of the transformation	Examine overlooked adaptive responses and adequately evaluate and integrate them	Replace the problem plot with a revised plot containing unique outcomes
Responsibility	Therapeutic climate establishes person as own agent and practitioner as agent of occupational environments	Personal authorship of one's own life story allows for agency and personal preference
Cause	Adaptation stimulated by occupational challenge	Change precipitated by crisis
Key words	Adapt	Revise
Primary emphasis	Internal adaptation process	Revision
Suggested primary sources	Schkade and Schultz (1992), Schultz and Schkade (1992)	Doan (1997), Parry and Doan (1994), Polkinghorne (1996)

Note. OA = occupational adaption.

occupational therapy. Situated on an academic health center campus, the program admits 32 junior students each fall into a sequenced full-time curriculum. At the time of this student's experience, the second semester of study posed the greatest challenge to students. The 16-credit hour semester consisted of 7 credit hours in 2 rigorous basic science courses, neurobiology and pathology. Before changes in the neurobiology course, between 2% and 5% of physical therapy and occupational therapy students earned grades of D in neurobiology on their first attempt, and some students dropped the course with grades of D or F. Most students took the course the next year, and a second grade of D or F resulted in dismissal from the program. Students perceived the spring semester to be challenging and placed special emphasis on passing the science-based courses.

The Student's Story

Mary (her chosen assumed name for this article) was admitted to the program shortly after her 22nd birthday. She had an entering cumulative grade point average (GPA) of 3.813 and a science GPA of 3.851. Mary had a bright affect, winning personality, and a strong religious faith that she related easily in conversation. Proclaiming one's spirituality, faith, and religious beliefs through discussion, clothing, and jewelry is an accepted part of the state's culture. Working in a public institution on an academic health center campus, I let students bring up topics that I might initiate if I were teaching on a private, religiously affiliated, or liberal arts campus.

Like most of her peers, Mary had never experienced academic failure, although she admitted that she "had to work harder than others." In the first semester of the occupational therapy program, she earned a GPA of 3.48; her lowest grade was a C in a rigorous kinesiology course. In the second semester, Mary's occupational challenge was to pass the neurobiology course with a grade of C or better. She was earning grades of B and C in two other science courses and simultaneously planning her December wedding to a physical therapy senior student. She planned to begin her Level II fieldwork placement in January. Mary discussed her frustration about long hours of studying and failing test scores with several other faculty members. She came to me for help during spring break, when she was on campus helping to interview applicants for admission.

After a brief discussion, it was apparent that Mary had incorporated all of the study and test-taking strategies recommended the previous semester. Having made scores of 60, after "a month of studying," and 71 on the first two neurobiology examinations, Mary placed extraordinary expectations on herself to pass the next two tests and the comprehensive final examination. Her fiancé and other study partners kept telling her that she "*knew* this stuff." However, something *was* new. Mary described thoughts of failure that interfered with studying for and taking neurobiology tests. She described her negative internal dialogue about her academic inadequacies and her mother's prediction that "fear always gets me on the first test." She told of a repeated vision of failure in which she saw a failing grade posted next to her name on a bulletin board. She said she hunched over the test with shaking hands, a nauseous stomach, and a pounding heart. She tried to use her faith but had squeezed a Christian cross so hard during the last examination that she hurt her hand.

Evaluation

In OA terms, Mary's problem lay within the adaptive response generation sub-process. Of the three components, Mary used the primary type of adaptation energy to study for and take tests, not shunting to the more sophisticated, creative, and less tiring secondary type of adaptation energy. She spent her primary energy in worry and task-irrelevant behavior. She used an existing mode of adaptive responses rather than using modified or new modes for study or taking tests. Mary's adaptive response behavior was hyperstabilized or stuck in repeating primitive patterns, such as imagining failure experiences. All three components combined to produce an adaptation gestalt that featured high psychosocial involvement and resulted in the sensorimotor symptoms of anxiety. Mary had high cognitive involvement directed to task-irrelevant thoughts and low involvement in task-relevant ones.

Within the adaptive response evaluation subprocess, Mary evaluated her relative mastery in studying for and taking examinations. She rated her mastery as low in effectiveness for not passing the tests, low in efficiency for the time and energy spend studying and achieving poor results, and low in personal satisfaction with her scores combined with embarrassment about her academic failure. Along the OA continuum with OA on one end, homeostasis in the middle, and occupational dysadaptation at the other, she evaluated herself as being dysadaptive. Within the adaptive response integration subprocess, Mary continually integrated her state of dysadaptation. She needed to generate at least one alternative adaptive response to enact, evaluate, and integrate.

In narrative terms, Mary was so dominated by her story of failure that she could not generate new stories with improved endings. She was stuck in a victim's problem-saturated plot, unable to generate alternative stories. Mary's submersion into the problem-saturated plot of failure led her to identity herself as the problem in a new role of "failing student." She was acting out a story of student failure.

Mary's occupational challenge required that she adapt and revise the story of failure to one with an improved ending. Transforming her story about the course had the potential to change her life story from one of failure to one of success. She could change the story and, thus, adapt. She could adapt and, thus, revise the story. The problem she faced was test anxiety specific to the neurobiology course, and the next examination was a month away.

Intervention

The deconstruction of Mary's problem plot created space for adaptation. We identified fear, not Mary, as the problem. Speaking to her of Fear, Trouble, Frustration, Pressure, and Doubt as characters in her problem plot, it seemed that Trouble had entered her academic life by using Frustration, Pressure, and Doubt to cause conflict. I shared my perspective that Fear was tricking her to fail academically. It seemed that Fear had even perverted the meaning of the Christian cross by making it hurt her. I wondered aloud how much more of her academic life she was willing to hand over to Fear. Mary readily agreed and externalized Fear as a gray and mist-like being. Once relieved of being the problem and enacting the role of failing student, Mary began the revision of her story through the internal adaptation process.

To begin the revision process, I pointed out unique outcomes that Mary had casually disregarded in their submersion by the problem plot. By evoking her overlooked adaptive responses, we calculated that she had passed approximately 115 examinations up to this point, noted that she had been accepted into a highly competitive academic program, and considered that she had passed the second examination in the first-semester kinesiology course after having failed the first one. She was surprised to hear me say that she was passing two other science-based courses that semester. Her face lit up with amazement at these realizations because the problem plot was so strong.

By asking Mary to tell me what made her think she would be a good occupational therapy practitioner in the first place, she enthusiastically told her story of preference, that of being an occupational therapy practitioner and being married. By literally writing out features of the problem plot and the preferred plot side by side on a large sheet of paper, Mary began to locate thoughts, feelings, and actions as belonging in one story or the other. Through narrative, Mary could vicariously envision and evaluate several alternative adaptive responses. We then began work on the constraints that kept Mary living out the problem and removed from her preferences.

For contrast with Fear, I asked her how Love would study, take an examination, and look at her posted scores. Her face softened as she articulated the newly generated adaptive response by saying, "Love would tell me 'I still love you' and I'd see a positive score. I'd talk with God before the test and relax." When I asked how that might work, her face was suddenly transformed, beaming with delight mixed with surprise, and she said, "All I ever had to do was turn it over to the Lord." I asked her to name a safe place where she could put Fear during the next examination so it would not bother her. Ignoring my suggestion, she breezily said she would "leave it with the Lord" and left my office radiating confidence. I shared her elation but worried that her reliance on faith might mean that she would no longer study. My own fear was unfounded and short-lived.

Outcomes

A few days later, Mary reported that she'd made a score of 92 on the third examination. She scored a 93 on the fourth, and a 90 on the comprehensive final examination. She made a B in the course and finished the semester with a GPA of 3.125.

Almost two semesters later, I asked Mary about this process. She said that talking to me during our two 45-min sessions "helped her some." She primarily credited prayer and her mother giving her supportive Bible verses to remind her that "God put you in this program for a reason." The change in her mother's behavior shows that Mary was able to recruit support for her preferred plot (Doan, 1997) and signaled adaptation as a result of the evaluation response and incorporation of adaptation (Schkade & Schultz, 1992) in her social and cultural occupational environments. Mary said she had a sense that God wanted her to succeed, so she had restructured her negative thought patterns by saying "Quit telling yourself that—it's not going to happen" and "Just shut up" when overcome with doubt and anxiety. She rated her ability to take other examinations as high in effectiveness, efficiency, and satisfaction.

Discussion

In deciding to use a narrative approach, I chose not to apply more traditional interventions from occupational therapy and education. Mary's story could easily lend itself to traditional intervention or explicit education on occupational therapy theory. For example, we could have crafted a container for Fear. However, Mary had no need to experience the rituals of either containment or release. Her faith led her to expect that God would remove Fear on her request through prayer. Another traditional medium, the progressive practice of skill until independent, would have been similarly ineffective. Mary was already applying the study and test-taking skills learned the previous semester. Insistence on a tangible product could have interfered with her process of internal OA. Mary's internal adaptation process needed to change, not be contained, released, or practiced.

In my role as educator, I could have explicitly approached Mary's problem as an example of OA theory. However, I sensed this could confuse the issue. We could have explored recent occupational therapy literature on spirituality, but Mary seemed certain that her self-doubt was a doubt of her faith and that prayer was her answer.

By using OA to guide the therapeutic climate (Schultz & Schkade, 1992), I allowed Mary to function as her own agent while I represented her occupational environments. I viewed my primary role as occupational therapy academician and advisor, not as provider of personal counseling or psychotherapy, neither of which I am qualified to do. Momentarily, I relinquished the opportunity to further her education about occupational therapy theory. As a result of my consideration of our roles, I left her story as story.

In preserving her challenge in narrative form, I honored the narrative truth as Mary told it. I privileged her voice (Doan, 1997) by keeping her truth in a form that made sense to her. By approaching her challenge as story, I listened and invited her to examine and revise it within the narrative metaphor she presented. In doing so, we worked in a medium familiar to all humans as natural storytellers.

Mary's story illustrates the many reasons humans tell stories. Mary needed to tell and retell her story, and she needed me, as an aspect of her social and cultural environment, to react to it (Frank, 1995). We use narrative as the agent by which we construct and reconstruct identity (McAdams, 1993; Polkinghorne, 1996). Mary's story showed her refusal of a new identity as a failing student. Humans tell stories to give or revise meanings of our experience (Bruner, 1990; Doan, 1997; Polkinghorne, 1996). Mary changed the meaning of her admission into the program as evidence of God's will for her life, one she could not easily revoke by failing a course. We tell stories to organize experience (Bruner, 1990) and bring cohesion to disparate actions (Mattingly, 1991; Polkinghorne, 1996), as Mary did when she linked her symptoms of anxiety to the tests in the course. We tell stories about unusual, not ordinary, events (Bruner, 1990). The fact that Mary formulated her experiences into story form indicated that academic failure was outside her usual experience. Mary clearly used story to link proposed actions to accomplish goals (Mattingly, 1991; Polkinghorne, 1996). Because every storyteller must have a story listener, we tell stories to observe the reaction of listeners and to verify our truth by seeing it reflected by someone else (Frank, 1995). Mary told me her story, anticipating that I would view her academic problems as uncharacteristic and share her distress.

Mary's eagerness to discuss her challenge in story affirmed my decision to use the narrative format. When discussing Fear as a character, I asked her if I were talking differently than I usually did. She denied that I was "talking funny" to her, further affirming its use. With silence as the only alternative to telling stories (Parry & Doan, 1994), Mary knew her continued silence would not help her pass the course.

Although Mary's story clearly illustrated several of the most characteristic features of test anxiety (Barnes, 1987; Everson, 1993; Frierson & Hoban, 1992; Howell & Swanson, 1989; Poorman, 1988; Poorman & Martin, 1991; Waltman, 1992), we collaborated on an intervention not discussed in that literature. The intervention worked and was entirely consistent with OA (Schkade & Schultz, 1992; Schultz & Schkade, 1992), the profession's grounding in the use of narrative as a therapeutic tool, and the narrative metaphor.

The narrative facilitation of adaptation itself was occupational. OA defines occupation as activity in which the person actively participates in a meaningful process, which results in a tangible or intangible product (Schkade & Schultz, 1992). Our discussion fits the definition of occupation as an active, meaningful activity that resulted in an intangible, verbal product. Given our roles as professor and student, a verbal product was appropriate and expected. The academic roles in Mary's story reminded me of Clark's (1993) discussions about occupation with Richardson that she called "occupational storytelling" and "occupational story making" (p. 1067). Noting that these methods "can become the core of [occupational therapy] clinical practice" (p. 1067), Clark (1993) pointed out that the mere telling of the person's story centered on occupation can be "enormously therapeutic" (p. 1068). As their discussions grew from research into occupational therapy, Clark said "it soon became clear that I had begun to function as her occupational therapist, through encouraging her to tell her story and by helping her to imagine new possibilities" (1993, p. 1073). Clark's synopsis could likewise describe the verbal exchange that Mary and I shared.

The focus of the OA frame of reference is the person's internal adaptation process (Schkade & Schultz, 1992; Schultz & Schkade, 1992), not the pursuit of skill or independence in skilled performance. By allowing Mary to adapt and discover her own method of stopping irrelevant thoughts, I furthered her internal adaptation. Although OA supports necessary skill-based intervention (Schultz & Schkade, 1992), Mary did not need to learn or practice them; further skill-based intervention would have diverted Mary from her need for internal adaptation.

Conclusion

As academic and clinical educators, we have numerous opportunities to facilitate students' adaptation and clinical reasoning. The comparison of two opposing plots or scenarios suggests further application. Students could contrast the use of two theories and their evaluation and intervention methods for a patient. We could ask them to compare interventions and outcomes for two clients with similar conditions. Students could consider the effect of two treatment environments for a client. The possibilities for application are limited only by the challenges faced by students in classroom or clinical settings.

In Mary's case, the synergy of the three theoretical bases contributed to a positive outcome. Her internal adaptation allowed her to meet the occupational challenge with relative mastery. Mary experienced OA by generating new adaptive responses that were self-initiated, generalized, and resulted in high degrees of effectiveness, efficiency, and satisfaction (Schkade & Schultz, 1992). She allowed her narrative to provide improved options and inform her choices (Clark et al., 1996; Larson & Fanchiang, 1996a; Mattingly, 1991; Polkinghorne, 1996). She transformed her plot from that of a victim to that of an agent of change (Polkinghorne, 1996). Mary deconstructed the problem plot and created a revision of her story (Doan, 1997; Parry & Doan, 1994). Through the synergy formed by the three bases of the intervention, Mary told herself a new story in adaptive language and created a happy ending. ▪

Acknowledgment

The author gratefully acknowledges the contribution of Dr. Robert E. Doan in the appreciation of the narrative metaphor.

References

American Occupational Therapy Association. (1979). The philosophical base of occupational therapy. *American Journal of Occupational Therapy, 33*, 785.

Barnes, R. G. (1987). Test anxiety in master's students: A comparative study. *Journal of Nursing Education, 26,* 12–19.

Bruner, J. (1990). *Acts of meaning.* Cambridge, MA: Harvard University Press.

Clark, F. (1993). Occupation embedded in a real life: Interweaving occupational science and occupational therapy. *American Journal of Occupational Therapy, 47*, 1067–1078.

Clark, F., Ennevor, B., & Richardson, P. (1996). A grounded theory of techniques for occupational storytelling and occupational story making. In R. Zemke & F. Clark (Eds.), *Occupational science: The evolving discipline* (pp. 373–392). Philadelphia: F. A. Davis.

Cohn, E. S. (1991). Special issue on clinical reasoning [Special issue]. *American Journal of Occupational Therapy, 45*(11).

Doan, R. E. (1997). *Narrathings: Guidelines for narrative therapy.* Unpublished manuscript, University of Oklahoma and Rogers University, Tulsa, OK.

Everson, H. T. (1993). *Test anxiety and the curriculum: The subject matters.* (Educational Resources Information Center documents). Bethesda, MD: ERIC Document Reproduction Service.

Frank, A. W. (1995). *The wounded storyteller: Body, illness, and ethics.* Chicago: University of Chicago Press.

Frierson, H. T. Jr., & Hoban, J. D. (1992). The effects of acute test anxiety on NBME Part I performance. *Journal of the National Medical Association, 84*, 686–689.

Helfrich, C., & Kielhofner, G. (1994). Volitional narratives and the meaning of therapy. *American Journal of Occupational Therapy, 48*, 319–326.

Helfrich, C., Kielhofner, G., & Mattingly, C. (1994). Volition as narrative: Understanding motivation in chronic illness. *American Journal of Occupational Therapy, 48*, 311–317.

Howell, C. C., & Swanson, S. C. (1989). The relative influence of identified components of test anxiety in baccalaureate nursing students. *Journal of Nursing Education, 28*, 215–220.

Larson, E. A., & Fanchiang, S. C. (1996a). Nationally Speaking—Life history and narrative research: Generating a humanistic knowledge base for occupational therapy. *American Journal of Occupational Therapy, 50*, 247–250.

Larson, E. A., & Fanchiang, S. C. (1996b). Special issue on life history and narrative in clinical practice [Special issue]. *American Journal of Occupational Therapy, 50*(4).

Mallinson, T., Kielhofner, G., & Mattingly, C. (1996). Metaphor and meaning in a clinical interview. *American Journal of Occupational Therapy, 50*, 338–346.

Mattingly, C. (1991). The narrative nature of clinical reasoning. *American Journal of Occupational Therapy, 45,* 998–1005.

McAdams, D. P. (1993). *The stories we live by: Personal myths and the making of the self.* New York: Morrow.

Parry, A., & Doan, R. E. (1994). *Story re-visions: Narrative therapy in the postmodern world.* New York: Guilford.

Polkinghorne, D. E. (1996). Transformative narrative: From victimic to agentic life plots. *American Journal of Occupational Therapy, 50,* 299–305.

Poorman, S. G. (1988). *Levels of test anxiety and cognitions of second semester senior level baccalaureate nursing students preparing for licensure exam* [Abstract]. Unpublished manuscript, University of Pittsburgh, Pittsburgh, PA.

Poorman, S. G., & Martin, E. J. (1991). The role of nonacademic variables in passing the National Council Licensure Examination. *Journal of Professional Nursing, 7,* 25–32.

Schkade, J., & Schultz, S. (1992). Occupational adaptation: Toward a holistic approach for contemporary practice: Part 1. *American Journal of Occupational Therapy, 46,* 829–837.

Schultz, S., & Schkade, J. (1992). Occupational adaptation: Toward a holistic approach for contemporary practice: Part 2. *American Journal of Occupational Therapy, 46,* 917–925.

Waltman, P. A. S. (1992). *Assessment of a test anxiety model with traditional and nontraditional students nurses* [Abstract]. Unpublished manuscript, University of Southern Mississippi, Hattiesburg.

Student Experiences in Multicultural Pediatric Settings

Karin J. Barnes

Gale Haradon

Nancy Hudepohl

Ida Garcia

Douglas Murphy

Karin J. Barnes, MS, OTR, is Associate Professor, Gale Haradon, PhD, OTR, is Associate Professor, Nancy Hudepohl, PhD, is Educational Development Specialist, Ida Garcia is Testing Center Coordinator, and Douglas Murphy, PhD, is Evaluation Specialist, The University of Texas Health Science Center at San Antonio, San Antonio, Texas. This work was supported by a grant from the Health Education Training Centers in Alliance of Texas (HETCAT), San Antonio, Texas.

The purpose of this project was to determine the effects of exposure to multicultural pediatric community settings to increase understanding of strategies that encourage students to consider community pediatric employment. Thirty-five senior occupational therapy students enrolled in a developmental theory and skills course attended an initial cultural diversity workshop. They were assigned to 1 of 8 groups to participate in evaluation and intervention programs for children with disabilities attending Headstart community programs. Preproject, midpoint, and post-project scores of the students' level of anxiety, general feelings of concern, and presence of preconceived stereotypes were measured. Experiences with Headstart children during an academic course was an effective strategy in decreasing student anxiety and facilitating the development of positive attitudes toward working in unfamiliar community settings. Recurrent cultural awareness workshops are suggested to have a greater effect than one initial orientation before the students' exposure to the community.

G RADUATES FROM THE OCCUPATIONAL THERAPY DEPARTMENT at The University of Texas Health Science Center at San Antonio (UTHSCSA) rarely sought employment in the regional multicultural pediatric community settings from 1989 to 1995. Only 2 out of 161 graduates accepted positions in community pediatric settings during this time. Most UTHSCSA occupational therapy graduates were initially employed in more traditional adult settings such as hospitals and rehabilitation centers. The UTHSCSA faculty members sought to develop strategies to encourage students to consider pediatric occupational therapy employment in the multicultural community.

The occupational therapy faculty members believed there were several curricular reasons that contributed to this problem. First, the occupational therapy program had not been able to provide the students with adequate experience in multicultural pediatric community settings in this region. This appeared to be related to immense didactic requirements for covering disability categories, theoretical and practical components of occupational therapy intervention, related medical interventions, and a need for exposure to the acute and chronic settings of hospitals and nursing homes. Little exposure was given to pediatric intervention in the context of the community, despite the faculty members' commitment to this area of practice. Consequently, students may have been more at ease in traditional medical adult settings.

Second, within the specific pediatric courses, exposure to young children with disabilities in natural school and community settings was limited due to scheduling and other constraints. The pediatric occupational therapy courses included didactic content of evaluation and treatment procedures for deficits in sensorimotor, oral motor, cognitive behavioral, positioning, prehension, activities of daily living, school performance, and prevocational skills. Pediatric service delivery, collaborative team approach, and pediatric documentation were discussed, but this did not allow sufficient exposure to children with disabilities within their environmental context that would decrease possible student fears about this practice area. Additionally, student confidence and interest in pediatric community intervention were not developed.

Last, past experience showed that finding clinical community experiences with pediatric patients was difficult due to several reasons. Observations and handling of young children often occur only with small groups of students (2 to 3), unlike adult settings, which may allow 6 to 10 students. Frequently, administrators at pediatric centers would not allow close observations and interactions with the young clients out of a protective concern for the children. Additionally, pediatric settings in San Antonio are dispersed throughout the large metropolitan area, which makes student access difficult. Without the "hands-on" evaluation and intervention experience with children with disabilities in their natural settings, occupational therapy students could not understand or appreciate the many factors that influence community pediatric practice.

For these reasons, the occupational therapy faculty members decided to explore means by which occupational therapy students would have exposure to community pediatric settings. Coincidentally, the agency that administers the Headstart program in San Antonio (Parent-Child, Inc.) contacted one of the occupational therapy faculty members and requested occupational therapy services for children with disabilities at Headstart centers throughout the city. The UTHSCSA Occupational Therapy Department agreed to provide these services, and occupational therapy students were allowed to observe and assist the occupational therapy faculty members. This would allow students to participate in the Headstart intervention as part of their existing pediatric occupational therapy course work. The much-needed exposure to children and family members of diverse cultural background, as well as children and family members of low socioeconomic status, would be possible.

Purpose of the Project

The purpose of this project was to provide an educational experience by which occupational therapy students could develop an appreciation and understanding for pediatric occupational therapy intervention with children and family members with culturally diverse backgrounds and low socioeconomic status. Specifically, the purpose was to determine the effects of exposure to multicultural pediatric community settings on students' levels of anxiety, general feelings of concern, and presence of preconceived stereotypes. The information would heighten awareness of strategies designed to encourage students to consider community pediatric employment.

Method

This project was designed to explore means by which to expose occupational therapy students enrolled in a developmental disabilities course to occupational therapy practice in multicultural settings with young children who attended San Antonio Headstart programs. The students were assigned to 1 of 8 groups that participated in the evaluation and intervention programs of children with disabilities attending Headstart programs. Preproject, midpoint, and postproject scores of the students' levels of anxiety, general feelings of concern, and presence of preconceived stereotypes were measured.

Participants

The participants were 35 senior occupational therapy students who were enrolled in developmental occupational therapy theory and skills courses at UTHSCSA. The diversity composition of the students was 27 white, 5 Mexican-American, and 3 Asian-American.

Instrumentation

There were four measurements of this project as described below. The first three were used before the interventions, at a midpoint in the project, and at the completion of the project. The last measurement, student comments, was completed at the end of the project.

Level of Anxiety

Level of student anxiety was measured because the faculty members believed that anxiety about experiences in community multicultural pediatric settings could be present. To investigate the relationship between participation in the community-based program and students' anxiety, the State-Trait Anxiety Inventory by Spielberger (1983) was administered after the program orientation, 9 days after students had begun their interventions, and at the end of the semester. Items related to trait anxiety were only used after the program orientation to determine if these students were different from the norm group in anxiety proneness.

The inventory consists of 20 items that measure a transitory condition of perceived tension. The form consists of 20 items that measure a relatively stable condition of anxiety proneness. Alpha reliability coefficients for the normative samples (high-school juniors, college freshmen, introductory psychology students) range from 0.83 to 0.92 for state scores and from 0.86 to 0.92 for trait scores. Validity coefficients for trait scores were estimated by correlating the scores with the Institute for Personality and Ability Testing

Anxiety Scale, Manifest Anxiety Scale, and Affect Adjective Check List (Spielberger, 1983). For 126 college women, coefficients were 0.75, 0.80, and 0.52, respectively.

Open-Ended Responses

Each occupational therapy student was asked to list what made them anxious about working with poor, culturally different children in community settings. After they listed these reasons, they were asked to rank the items, starting with 1 as the item that caused the most anxiety.

Bipolar Attractiveness Scale

Students were administered an 8-item Bipolar Attractiveness Scale developed by the third author, who is an educational development specialist at UTHSCSA. This scale was designed to measure the students' attitudes toward clients on the basis of the following characteristics.

- Low socioeconomic status
- African-American
- Service in a community setting
- Hispanic-American
- Culturally different
- White American
- Different primary language
- Asian-American

Students marked their opinions of the "attractiveness" of these characteristics on 7-point semantic differential scales anchored by the following adjective pairs: good–bad, valuable–worthless, and clean–dirty.

Student Comments

At the completion of the project, the students were asked to respond to the following statements, which were written and compiled anonymously.

- What I liked about the project
- What I disliked about the project
- What I learned from the project
- Would I recommend the project?

Intervention

There were two components to the intervention procedure. First, there was a community intervention orientation program provided by the UTHSCSA occupational therapy faculty members and educational development specialists. This program was designed to provide information about the specific occupational therapy assignment and general information about regional multicultural pediatric settings (Table 1). The students were provided with an orientation to their impending involvement in the occupational therapy intervention at the community Headstart programs. This orientation used slides and lecture materials about the multicultural community experience. This was immediately followed by a 3-hr presentation on cultural diversity, community placement, and low socioeconomic status.

Second, after the workshop, the students were assigned to 1 of 8 groups to work with a specific child with a disability at 1 of 5 Headstart settings. The students were instructed to develop a comprehensive program that would allow the integration of therapy evaluation and intervention factors with the ecological factors of the children's school and home settings. Additionally, they were instructed to develop means by which to collaborate with the child's teacher and parents.

The students accompanied the occupational therapy faculty members to the Headstart settings weekly to conduct evaluations, meet with teachers, and provide occupational therapy intervention. Additionally, the students met periodically with the faculty members to discuss the project. At the completion of the semester, the students handed in their notebooks for a course grade (Table 2). Copies of the classroom and home programs were provided for the teachers, and the students discussed these with the teachers in some cases.

Results

The results for the first 3 measures included 27 of 35 students. The excluded 8 students did not have data for all three measures across the 3 administrations. However, all 35 students completed the group intervention project.

Table 1
Student Learning Objectives

Occupational therapy students will demonstrate the following:

- Increased understanding and appreciation of diverse cultures
- An increased awareness of issues related to low socioeconomic status
- Beginning mastery in the administration of standardized assessments to young children with disabilities
- Beginning mastery in the writing of goals and objectives
- Critical problem-solving skills necessary to develop direct therapy, classroom, and home intervention programs
- Interpersonal skills with children, teachers, and parents

Table 2
Student Intervention Projects

■ Written evaluation results from the Peabody Developmental Motor Scale (Folio & Fewell, 1983)

■ Problem list (underlying developmental disabilities noted)

■ Importance of the disabilities in relation to home and school

■ Goal and objective list

■ Direct occupational therapy activities

■ Indirect classroom activities

■ Indirect home activities

■ Rationale for intervention activities

■ Documentation strategies

■ Reference sources used

State-Trait Anxiety Inventory

Trait anxiety. The 34.50 mean for men (n = 6) and 35.79 mean for women (n = 21) were tested against the means for the norm group of working adults 19 to 39 years of age (men = 35.55, women = 36.15). The z test showed no significant difference, meaning that this group of students was not inclined to anxiety any more than the norm group.

State anxiety. Applying the related measures analysis of variance (ANOVA) for "time" effect to the means reported for the State Anxiety Inventory (30.22, 33.37, and 28.07) did not indicate a significant effect [$F(2,52) = 3.21, p > 0.05$]. The ANOVA for trends revealed no significant linear trend but did reveal a significant quadratic trend [$F(1,52) = 5.38, p = 0.05$] (Table 3, Figure 1).

Open-Ended Responses

Students' open-ended responses were categorized, and responses to these categories across time were noted by percentage response (Table 4). Concerns that

Table 3
State Anxiety Inventory (ANOVA for "Time" and "Trend" Effect)

	Preproject	9 days	Postproject	Time Effect (F)	Trend (F)
Mean	30.22	33.37	28.07	3.21	Quadratic 5.38*
SD	9.24	13.08	7.81		

Note. *$p < 0.05$. *SD* = standard deviation.

were reported across the total rotation were communication (54%, 46%, 34%), culture (29%, 25%, 17%), and environment and safety (32%, 18%, 37%). Concerns reported that showed a decrease over time were knowledge and skill base (25%, 7%, 3%) and therapy (26%, 4%, 11%). Concerns reported only during the orientation program were affective dimension (6%), expectations (6%), poverty (19%), resources (3%), and supervision and evaluation (3%). Concerns reported for both the first and last session were clients (19%, 9%). Responses noted for "No concerns" occurred only in sessions 2 and 3 (36%, 29%).

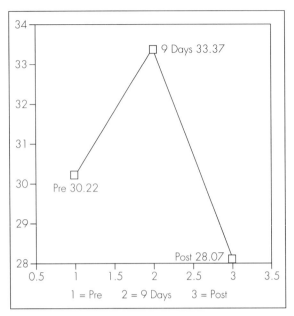

Figure 1. State anxiety means.

Bipolar Attractiveness Scale

A mean of the three bipolar adjectives was calculated for each of the eight characteristics. No significant difference was found for any of the characteristics across time. However, the ANOVA for trends revealed a significant linear trend in the means for low socioeconomic status [$F(1,52) = 4.17, p < 0.05$] and a significant quadratic trend in the means for community setting [$F(1,52) = 5.14, p < 0.05$].

Student Comments

Each student anonymously provided written feedback about the project. Here are some representative responses.

- "I liked the direct/hands-on experience that this project provided. I also enjoyed the experience of going to a Headstart facility and actually understanding the dynamics of this group. I felt the IEP [individualized education program] with the family present provided an excellent example for future employment atmospheres."

- "I liked being involved in the complete processes, the observations, evaluation, treatment development, and treatment intervention."

- "I learned that you must specifically tailor the OT intervention to the needs of the family and the child and the teacher."

- "[I disliked] trying to find the center and getting lost and being on time."

Table 4
Open-Ended Responses

	Preproject	%	Midpoint	%	Postproject	%
Affective dimension	2	6				
Clients	6	19			3	9
Communication	17	54	13	46	12	34
Culture	9	29	7	25	6	17
Environment and safety	10	32	5	18	13	37
Expectations	2	6				
Knowledge and skill base	8	25	2	7	1	3
Poverty	6	19				
Resources	1	3				
Supervision and evaluation	1	3				
Therapy	8	26	1	4	4	11
No concerns			10	36	10	9

Note. N = 31 for Preproject, N = 28 for Midpoint, N = 29 for Postproject.

■ "[I disliked] scheduling."

■ "I learned therapy can be in all different settings."

■ "I did not like showing up and finding out the child was unavailable (but that was no one's fault)."

■ "I learned that there are not set formulas for treatment and that data collection is a key to good treatment planning."

■ "I didn't like the inordinate amount of time it took to do the treatment plan."

■ "I really enjoyed having the opportunity to work with a variety of cultures. I feel that I have become more aware of the wants, needs, and desires associated with other cultures."

■ "I did not like the [Bipolar Attractiveness Scale] because it is difficult to answer questions such as is an Anglo dirty or clean—that all depends on the person. I am very open minded, and I don't judge anyone because of their culture."

■ "I learned that children don't always behave as we have planned in our practice scenarios."

■ "Language in different cultures wasn't near the problem I thought it was."

The students then answered the question, "Would you recommend this project for other students?" Twenty-seven answered "yes," and 3 students answered "no" (due to time issues and the cultural workshop).

Discussion

Data reported for the State Anxiety Inventory indicated that, when students had no actual experience with the environment (preprogram), their anxiety levels were relatively low; but once they began working in the program for 9 days (initial immersion), their anxiety increased greatly. As they became more familiar with the environment and what was expected of them, their anxiety dropped once again. Traditional orientation programs are conducted on the basis of the assumption that anxiety levels will be highest when the total environment is unknown. These results suggest that initial contact in a new setting may provoke greater levels of anxiety. Thus, community intervention orientation programs may be more effective in reducing student anxiety when the instructional content is staggered across time.

Results from the open-ended comments show that students have different concerns across time and that this should be taken into consideration when designing the content of a community intervention orientation program. Specific comments suggest that appropriate topics for the initial session could include the following:

- The affective aspect: offering suggestions on how to avoid inappropriate emotional involvement with the client and cope with expected emotional reactions such as dealing with a feeling of anger when team members do not comply with treatment plans

- The performance expectations: outlining specific activities, level of performance expected across the experience, resources, duties, timelines, supervision, and evaluation

- The clients: understanding developmental disabilities, the range of treatment options available, cultural and ethnic composition, linguistic differences, cultural values related to physical disability, and realities related to the culture of poverty such as body odor, head lice, and communicable diseases

- The community: safe travel strategies in high-crime neighborhoods, safe parking, and tips on appropriate and inappropriate behavior

After students have had a week's experience in the community setting, scheduled debriefing sessions throughout the educational experience could focus on specific communication problems encountered and how these may be addressed. These problems include client and practitioner trouble spots that may be caused by cultural differences, affective responses to clients, and issues related to the environmental context.

Consistently high means on all items on the Bipolar Attractiveness Scale suggest that this test may have not been appropriate for this project. This indicates the difficulty of objectively measuring attitudes toward clients and perhaps attitudinal shifts can be better gauged by student behavior and personal report in debriefings. However, the significant linear trend in the means for low socioeconomic status suggests that contact over time triggers a positive trend in attitude toward this dimension and that the length of a rotation would influence changes in attitude. The significant quadratic trend in the means for community setting reflect the trend seen for the means in the State Anxiety Inventory, that is, a decrease in positive attitude was concomitant with an increase in the level of anxiety during initial contact with clients and the community environment, but this improved with time. Lack of significance in the means for any of the racial or ethnic variables indicates that values and norms associated with the "culture of poverty" may be of greater concern and importance to serving children in the community setting. Therefore, distinctions should be made in training between values and norms associated with poverty, which is true regardless of race and ethnicity, and those that are unique and distinct to evaluating care and complying with treatment for specific cultural groups.

After this class of students graduated, 4 of the 27 who graduated took initial employment in community pediatric settings. However, the actual relationship between the increased employment in community pediatric settings and this project cannot be implied due to other extraneous factors.

Conclusion

The results of this study generated new understanding of the relationship of exposure to multicultural pediatric community settings on student level of anxiety, general feelings of concern, and presence of preconceived stereotypes. The students were shown to have the most anxiety about their communication abilities, cultural issues, safety in the environment, and poverty.

Students initially were anxious about working in unfamiliar settings, but weekly exposure during the time of the one-semester course lessened their anxiety and appeared to create interest in working in the community pediatric environment. Student anecdotal comments established the students' enjoyment of the direct hands-on experience of being involved in the evaluation and treatment of children in the community settings. The strategy to systematically expose students to multicultural community settings during a course appears to be a positive method to decrease anxiety and to develop positive attitudes over time to unfamiliar community settings. Ongoing community intervention orientation programs and discussions of factors that arise during the community experience are suggested to have a greater value than one initial orientation program before the students' experiences in the community.

Student exposure to children in multicultural community settings during a course in developmental disabilities appears to be an effective strategy to encourage students to consider community pediatric employment. ∎

References

Folio, M., & Fewell, R. (1983). *Peabody Developmental Motor Scales and Activity Cards*. Chicago: Riverside.

Spielberger, C. D. (1983). *State-Trait Anxiety Inventory for Adults*. Palo Alto, CA: Mind Garden.

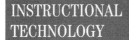
Internet Use by Occupational Therapy Education Programs

Theodore I. King, II

Theodore I. King, II, PhD, OT, is Associate Professor, Occupational Therapy Program, University of Wisconsin-Milwaukee, Milwaukee, Wisconsin.

Survey data were collected from a questionnaire mailed to all accredited occupational therapy educational programs (professional and technical levels) in the United States (N = 300). Information collected included: student access to the Internet on campus, faculty member use of e-mail to communicate with each other and with students, faculty member use of the World Wide Web, and program and institutional use of the World Wide Web for instructional purposes. Questionnaires were returned from 70% of the sample (n = 211). Responses from the survey indicated that 96% of students in these programs have campus access to the Internet, and more than 90% of occupational therapy programs currently use or plan to use the Internet for instructional purposes.

T HE INTERNET HAS BECOME A MAJOR INFORMATION-SHARING database. Persons of all ages are using the Internet as a means to share or retrieve data and communicate with others. The Internet is a worldwide network infrastructure that allows data sharing between computers. The Internet has attracted major attention as a means of delivering instruction for two reasons.

1. Institutions may offer courses to students worldwide because campus "boundaries" are not confined to geographical limits

2. Pedagogical advantages exist in offering instruction via the Internet

Research on instructional delivery modes has shown that students learn better via distance education than with traditional classroom instruction (Moore, 1989). Although many institutions of higher education are instituting use of the Internet to increase enrollments, there are advantages for persons who have economic or transportation constraints, are working, or are single parents to be able to take courses via the Internet that offer the student choice of location and time.

A glossary of terms (Table 1) is included in this article to assist the reader with terms related to distance education and the potential instructional applications of the Internet. These applications provide diverse options to choose on the basis of one's learning objectives.

Purpose of the Study

This study was designed to collect and disseminate data related to the current use of the Internet by occupational therapy educational programs throughout the United States. The following eight questions regarding access and use of the Internet were developed and included in the survey.

1. Do students in your program have campus access to the World Wide Web?

Table 1
Glossary of Terms

- *Asynchronous instruction:* a distance education delivery mode allowing students to individually choose their own instructional time and place. Initially, the most common form of asynchronous instruction was correspondence courses that included the use of audio-cassettes and videotapes. Recently, the Internet has become a common form of asynchronous instruction by using e-mail, listservs, and the World Wide Web.

- *Distance education:* refers to offering courses in a way that does not require the student to be in the same location as the instructor.

- *E-mail:* a means of communicating with millions of people via the Internet. In a course, e-mail allows students to communicate with each other, the instructor, and experts in the field.

- *Internet:* a worldwide network infrastructure that allows data sharing between computers. Educational uses of the Internet include e-mail, listservs, and the World Wide Web.

- *Listserv:* an electronic mailing list used for group discussions. A person on a listserv will receive all e-mail sent to the list and may participate by sending a response that will be received by all listserv members.

- *Synchronous instruction:* a distance education delivery mode where the instructor and all students participate simultaneously (e.g., videoconferencing).

- *Uniform resource locator (URL):* a naming scheme for locating Internet resources. By using an Internet browser (e.g., Netscape™ [Netscape Communications Corporation, Mountain View, CA] or Microsoft Internet Explorer™ [Microsoft Corporation, Redmond, WA]), the URL or Internet address may be entered to go to a specific resource.

- *World Wide Web:* allows users to access Internet information containing text files, graphics, sounds, and videos located at a specific Internet address or URL.

2. Do faculty members in your program use e-mail to communicate with each other?

3. Do faculty members in your program use e-mail to communicate with students?

4. Do faculty members in your program access the World Wide Web for work-related reasons?

5. Is the World Wide Web used by your institution for instructional purposes?

6. Is the World Wide Web used by your program for instructional purposes?

7. If your program does not currently use the World Wide Web for instructional purposes, are there plans to do so in the future?

8. Do you believe a course on the World Wide Web offers the same quality of instruction as classroom teaching?

Methods

The study sample consisted of all accredited occupational therapy educational programs (professional and technical levels) in the United States. The list of program directors and schools was received from the American Occupational Therapy Association and totaled 300 (133 occupational therapy programs and 167 occupational therapy assistant programs). The survey was designed to be completed by the program director, and each question was answered "yes" or "no" to expedite completion of the survey and enhance returns. The surveys were mailed to the sample along with self-addressed stamped envelopes. Recipients were requested to complete and return the survey within 4 weeks.

Results

Surveys were returned from 94 occupational therapy programs (71%) and 117 occupational therapy assistant programs (70%). Results were tabulated for each of the questions in the survey to indicate percentage of the respondents answering "yes" versus "no." Because this is a descriptive survey study rather than experimental or methodological, data and statistical analyses are not appropriate to determine significance and are not included. The percentage responding "yes" to each of the survey questions is represented in Figure 1

Students in both occupational therapy and occupational therapy assistant programs generally have access to the Internet (96%). E-mail is used less often in assistant programs between faculty members and students. All occupational therapy programs and 91% of occupational therapy assistant programs currently use or plan to use the World Wide Web for instructional purposes. Only 33% of all respondents indicated that they believed instruction via the Internet offers the same quality as classroom instruction, but many noted that quality may depend on the type of course being offered (e.g., lecture material vs. laboratory experiences).

Discussion

The major aim of this study was to determine the availability and use of the Internet in occupational therapy educational programs (professional and technical levels). The survey indicated that most campuses with occupational therapy programs offer Internet access to students and faculty members. Faculty members in professional programs tend to use the Internet more than faculty members in technical programs. This may reflect a difference in 4-year versus 2-year institutions and job requirements of faculty members. Overall, the survey indicated that 82% of institutions with occupational therapy programs (professional and technical levels) use the Internet for instructional purposes, but only 55% of the occupational therapy programs use the Internet for instructional purposes. This probably is due to greater emphasis on alternative teaching modes

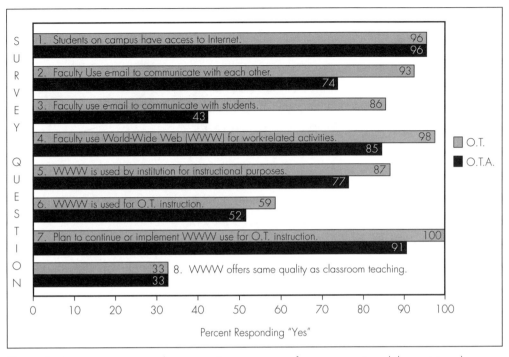

Figure 1. Internet survey results comparing responses from occupational therapist and occupational therapy assistant programs.

in other programs such as education and computer sciences. However, 95% of the occupational therapy programs indicated that they have plans to use the Internet for instructional purposes in the near future. This indicates the trend toward greater use of the Internet for instruction with e-mail (Boettcher, 1997; Zimmerman, 1998) and the World Wide Web (Ehrmann, 1995).

An example of current use of the World Wide Web for teaching purposes in an occupational therapy program is the Introduction to Occupational Therapy course offered at the University of Wisconsin–Milwaukee. This course is designed to introduce students to the field of occupational therapy before admission to the professional program. The course is taught primarily on the World Wide Web. Students come to class only for discussion and test-taking purposes. This course may be viewed at the following Web address: www.uwm.edu/~tking.

Summary

The Internet is a worldwide information-sharing database becoming popular as a means of delivering distance education (Willis, Robin, & Willis, 1995). The Internet includes e-mail, listservs, and the World Wide Web. Using the Internet for instructional purposes does not limit an institution to geographical boundaries, allows students choice of time and place, and has been shown to have pedagogical value. E-mail and listservs may be helpful in sharing program and course information within an occupational therapy program. Greater instructor accessibility and enhancement of course discussions are advantages to using these media. The World Wide Web allows students to view text files, graphics, sounds, and videos on an occupational therapy program's Web site for informational or educational purposes and may serve as a rich resource for specific course topics.

A survey of occupational therapy and occupational therapy assistant programs indicates wide access to the Internet with plans to increase its use for educational purposes. Rather than substituting computer-based or Internet teaching for other modes of instruction in an occupational therapy program, it may be most helpful to use the Internet as a supplement to lecture and laboratory experiences. Student interaction with the instructor and other students may be fostered through the use of technology (Berger, 1998). ▪

References

Berger, C. (1998). The four myths of integrating technology into teaching. *Syllabus, 11*, 18–20.

Boettcher, J. (1997). Internet pitfalls: What not to do when communicating with students on the Internet. *Syllabus, 11*, 46–52.

Ehrmann, S. C. (1995). Moving beyond campus-bound education. *Chronicle of Higher Education, 41*, A14.

Moore, M. (Ed.). (1989). *Readings in distance learning and instruction*. University Park, PA: Pennsylvania State University.

Willis, D., Robin, B., & Willis, J. (Eds.). (1995). *Technology and teacher education annual*. Charlottesville, VA: Association for Advancement of Computing in Education.

Zimmerman, S. (1998). Bringing electronic mail into the classroom: Teaching strategies. *Writing Across the Curriculum Newsletter, 8*, 1–3.

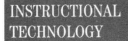

INSTRUCTIONAL
TECHNOLOGY

Peer Review of Teaching for Summative and Formative Evaluation in Occupational Therapy

Michael B. Worrell

Janet Everly

Celestine Hamant

Judith Kiel

Michael B. Worrell, PhD, is Assistant Professor, Janet Everly, MS, OTR, is Associate Professor, Celestine Hamant, MS, OTR, is Associate Professor and Program Director, and Judith Kiel, MS, OTR, is Clinical Associate Professor, Occupational Therapy Program, Indiana University School of Allied Health Sciences, Indianapolis, Indiana.

Teaching effectiveness has traditionally been evaluated through student evaluations and faculty review. The advent of new and innovative ways of teaching and an increasing concern for student outcomes calls for additional tools for evaluation of teaching to supplement the existing repertoire. We will present some of the process and results of peer review in the Occupational Therapy Program at Indiana University (IU) School of Allied Health Sciences. In this program, the faculty members are dedicated to teaching, and the environment is rich for peer review. The variety in the IU occupational therapy peer review process will be presented by using Hutchings' menu as a framework. Last, we will present a case study of external peer review of teaching that was intended to simulate the process of external peer review of research, which is frequently used but parallel to the external review process used for scholarship.

T EACHING EFFECTIVENESS HAS TRADITIONALLY BEEN EVALUATED through student evaluations and faculty review. Student evaluation of instruction has been a fixture in higher education for many years. Institutions have in their culture the practice of having classes observed by a senior faculty member or an administrator to evaluate a junior faculty member's performance. Some programs have all faculty members' classroom activities observed for content and style. With a shift in education to what Barr and Tagg (1995) called a *learning paradigm,* instructors produce learning with each student using whatever means works best. This teaching method has made student evaluations even more challenging. The advent of new and innovative ways of teaching and an increasing concern for student outcomes calls for additional tools for evaluation of teaching to supplement the existing repertoire. Review of teaching by peers in its many forms includes several effective means of evaluation.

Peer review is a natural consequence of a desire to improve or enhance one's teaching (Hutchings, 1995). The desire to evaluate one's teaching will often be led by two motivations.

1.   Formative evaluation
2.   Summative evaluation

Formative evaluation is evaluation with the purpose of improving content or style. *Summative evaluation* is evaluation with an administrative goal, which may include decisions of promotion, tenure, or retention. Both formative and summative evaluation are useful end products of peer review. It is important to note when one is being evaluated that the desired use of the information (i.e., formative or summative) be known to determine the method of evaluation or the format.

Teaching as a profession is looked on less favorably than research, in part, because teaching is not stringently evaluated (Seldin, 1993). Instructors at institutions where research is a component of academic life are familiar with the peer review process as applied to research. In these same institutions, teaching is often held in lower regard because it is less rigorously evaluated than research and because there are less tangible rewards for success in teaching. Peer review of teaching, when done properly, should elevate both the quality of instruction and the status of teaching within the academic environment.

Hutchings (1996) compiled a publication for the American Association of Higher Education that described "a menu for peer collaboration and peer review" (p. 3). This menu of nine options is the framework for this article. We will present some of the process and results of peer review in the Occupational Therapy Program at Indiana University (IU; Indianapolis, IN) School of Allied Health Sciences. In this program, the faculty members are dedicated to teaching, and the environment is rich for peer review. The variety in the IU occupational therapy peer review process will be presented by using Hutchings' menu as a framework. Last, we will present a case study of external peer review of teaching that was intended to simulate the process of external peer review of research, which is frequently used but parallel to the external review process used for scholarship.

Menu of Peer Review Options

In Hutchings' (1996) publication, nine general ideas are presented for conducting peer review. The need to use all of these forms of evaluation seldom occurs. Each option has its own merit and will be described along with what has been done in the IU program and the IU/Purdue University Indianapolis (IUPUI) campus.

Teaching Circles

Teaching circles (Bernstein, 1996) involve the participation of several instructors who meet to discuss particular teaching topics. The topic may be a point of discipline, specific content, pedagogical style, or a classroom problem. This means of evaluation allows for the initiation of conversation regarding teaching. The idea of teaching circles includes the regular participation of group members in this ongoing discussion. Once discussion is initiated, new topics can be added to supplement the conversation and to encourage problem solving of new issues.

In the IU program, the teaching circle is a weekly faculty meeting where topics of interest may be brought up for discussion. Student learning problems are discussed, and classroom techniques are tested on a willing and knowledgeable audience. This process ensures that the topic of teaching is always open for discussion with peers.

Reciprocal Visits and Observations

Classroom observation is the backbone of peer review. It is nonetheless intimidating to have a peer evaluating for weaknesses and strengths in content or style in one's classroom. By taking an active posture of inviting a peer into the classroom for formative evaluation, the fear of future summative evaluations may be alleviated. Having a visitor in the classroom allows the opportunity for more discussion on the topic of teaching.

A classroom observation is best done when there is a preobservation meeting to discuss the purpose of the observation and for the faculty member to explain the learning objectives for the session. This point is sometimes overlooked in the effort simply to fulfill the administrative requirement of having a peer review one's teaching.

Just as it is difficult for students to record and retain every aspect of what happens in a 50-min class period, an observer will have difficulty evaluating content, presentation, classroom interaction, and student reactions all at the same time. For a complete observation to take place, more than one visit may be required, or more than one observer may be invited. A standardized observation form or forms will facilitate the process by focusing what is desired from the observer.

Reciprocation is an ideal extension of the classroom visit. The shared experiences create a common bond that allows for further discussion and the possibility for collaboration on other endeavors. Care must be taken to form a context in which candid and constructive criticism can be shared. A clear set of goals and an understanding of the nature of the observation (formative vs. summative) helps to ensure openness. After any classroom visit, a postobservation meeting is essential for dissemination and perhaps interpretation of observation results.

Classroom observation has been a part of the IU program for many years. A fellow instructor is asked by the faculty member to visit a class to perform an observation. A standardized observation form that meets needs for accreditation has been developed by the IU program. Forms may need to be revised on the basis of the information desired from the observation. For example, the current form does not address small group facilitation. The existing form may be modified to address small group issues, or an entirely new form may be created. Pre- and postobservation meetings are held between the observer and the observee. Because of the small size of the program, reciprocal visits are the norm. The resultant observation and written comments are always used formatively and may be used summatively, especially for persons seeking tenure, promotion, or documentation for teaching recognition. Because of familiarity between faculty members, it is especially valuable to have outside reviewers make classroom observations. Recognized "style" experts or content experts from other departments have been used several times in this program.

Mentoring

Mentoring has deep roots in the history of apprenticing, where a senior or more experienced person guides the development of one less experienced. In teaching, the mentoring process has been established as part of the culture in many disciplines across the IUPUI campus. In some disciplines in which persons may have highly specialized knowledge and may not have a peer knowledgeable in a specific subject area, there may be a belief that mentoring cannot be achieved. The art and craft of teaching, although influenced by a discipline, is not necessarily dictated by discipline or subject. Another perceived difficulty is fear of inordinate time commitment on the part of the mentor. As with most activities involving a busy schedule, priorities and scheduling are keys to success with mentoring. Mentoring a developing teacher should be viewed as both a privilege and a challenge.

In the experience of this program, mentoring is not usually a one-on-one process. Because each person tends to have a specialty area, the rest of the experienced faculty members share thoughts, time, and resources with new faculty members. One faculty member who teaches students about teaching has prepared a handbook that is shared with all new faculty members that describes the basics of syllabus and test writing as well as overall course organization, including dealing with student issues and a format for paperwork. This veteran faculty member is available to consult with other faculty members.

Student Learning Outcomes

Just as a goal of peer review of teaching is to improve teaching and learning, student evaluation is critical to the process. Standardized course or instructor evaluation forms usually yield data concerning student perceptions and provide a common ground for comparison with other instructors. Course and instructor evaluations, especially written comments by the students, can guide changes in style or content that can help improve teaching and learning. When discussed with a knowledgeable colleague or colleagues, student evaluations can drive positive changes in instruction.

Teaching Portfolios

The teaching portfolio has become a powerful tool in documenting teaching. Seldin (1993) described a teaching portfolio as "...a factual description of a professor's teaching strengths and accomplishments." Some teaching portfolio proponents say that a portfolio must exist for each course taught, whereas others view the portfolio as a single document of a person's work. The content of a portfolio may vary but generally documents how and why the course is taught the way it is. Documentation of student work and other course artifacts are included for peer review. Often evidence of evaluation by peers is included in the portfolio to demonstrate that the course is appropriate for the audience and discipline (Davis & Swift, 1995). This documentation of peer review is of great value for most summative evaluations.

Although teaching portfolios are widely used on the IUPUI campus, the program has not initiated their use. A pilot project will begin with at least one of the instructors in the near future.

Team Teaching

Team teaching is commonplace in most institutions of higher education. In many instances, professor A will teach the first half of the course, and professor B will teach the second half. Start and stop points are agreed on by both. The content may be dictated by a discipline or text, but means of conveyance remains individualized. Team teaching that promotes peer review requires all of the members of the team to be involved in the preparation and execution of a course. Although it may be impractical for a team of six professors to be available for every class meeting of an individual course, they can each be involved in discussions concerning the course and foster a continuing dialogue on teaching and share the teaching workload.

Collaborative Inquiry

A theme that is recognized in peer review of teaching is establishing a dialogue among persons concerned about teaching. This mutual concern about teaching has the potential for facilitating alliances and collaborations that are capable of spawning scholarly works. The inquiry into ideas concerning teaching is often left to the realm of kindergarten to grade 12 teaching where Shulman (1989) and others have prepared the groundwork by which higher education peer review has flourished. As a pedagogical idea is explored, data can be collected to determine the effectiveness of changes and modifications to course content or presentation style. Collaborative inquiry in the IU program has lead to publication (Everly, Poff, Lamport, Hamant, & Alvey, 1994) and several manuscripts in preparation related to teaching and learning.

Departmental Occasions

When a department or program has the opportunity to have a presentation for its faculty members and perhaps students, the presentation will often reflect the interests of the program. Departmental (program) occasions can include presentations by candidates for teaching positions, in-service training opportunities, or invited lecturers. Because funds are limited for most facilities, it could be wise to put those limited resources to work supporting the important task of teaching. In-service presentations by visitors or faculty members can involve presentations about pedagogy, technology, or student evaluation. Research presentations can examine issues of interest to teaching or peer review.

Intercampus and External Review

In an initial foray into external peer review of teaching, Malik (1996) had faculty members put together written materials that were sent out for external reviews to peers in their specific discipline. Malik reported that, although the reviewers' analyses did not always address what was desired, the faculty members benefited from their own reflective analyses of their teaching.

Intercampus or external review of teaching is an infrequent activity seldom used in teaching review processes. However, this process parallels the typical external review process used for scholarship, which, as noted earlier, appears to be one of the factors making research more valued or prestigious. In the following pilot case study, a model to implement this unique process and its outcomes are described.

A Pilot Case Study of External Review

The IU program conducted a limited study of external peer review of teaching in Fall 1997. On the basis of the work by Malik (1996), a packet of information to evaluate the instructor was assembled by the occupational therapy peer review team, including printed materials received by the students in a specific course, an explanation of the goals of this external review (i.e., both formative and summative evaluation and evaluation for both style and content), and an explanation of the project. In addition, lectures in which the instructor was to be evaluated were videotaped and included in the packet for external reviewers.

The IU program director communicated with other program directors to ask for willing faculty members to evaluate this packet for both style and content. Two programs agreed to evaluate the teaching of one volunteer from the IU peer review team. Reviewers' comments were anonymously given in an effort to more closely simulate research evaluation. Only the IU program director was informed of the identities of the external reviewing institutions to promote candid appraisal. From the two external programs, three persons reviewed the packets and completed standardized evaluation forms. A fourth internal reviewer was solicited. Scores were ranked from 1 to 4, with 1 representing poor performance and 4 representing exemplary performance. The results of those evaluations are presented in Table 1. The evaluee, as a member of the peer review team, was immediately informed of the reviewers' scores and comments. The result was that the faculty members sought to make visual aids more visible throughout the room.

Discussion

Columns 1 through 3 of Table 1 represent the results from the three external reviewers, whereas the last column reflects the results of the internal reviewer. External reviewers' scores were consistently lower than those of the internal

Table 1
Results of Peer Review

| | Reviewers | | | | |
Criteria Evaluated by Reviewers	1	2	3	4	Average
1. Demonstrates knowledge of subject matter	4	4	4	4	4
2. Organizes subject matter clearly	4	4	3	4	3.75
3. Explains at audience's level	4	4	3	4	3.75
4. Encourages productive thinking (problem solving)	3	4	4	4	3.75
5. Demonstrates effective speaking skills	4	4	3	4	3.75
6. Stimulates audience participation	3	4	3.5	4	3.625
7. Responds well to audience feedback	4	4	3.5	4	3.875
8. Creates an atmosphere conducive to learning	4	4	4	4	4
9. Uses audiovisual materials to complement teaching	3	3	3	4	3.25
10. Takes a positive approach to audience	4	4	4	4	4
Total out of 40 possible points	37	39	35	40	37.75

Note. Reviewers 1 through 3 represent external reviewers, and 4 represents the internal reviewer. Scores are on a 1 to 4 scale with 1 = not fully competent, 2 = satisfactory, 3 = often exceeds normal requirements, and 4 = exemplary performance.

reviewer. Written comments collected from all of the reviewers reflected the same pattern. Differences in scores could be

▪ coincidental because this is a small pilot study, expected in that an internal reviewer would view his or her peer in a positive way or would be reluctant to document otherwise, or

▪ a reflection on the difference between viewing a videotape versus a live presentation.

For example, the internal reviewer commented specifically that the room limitations made effective use of visual aids difficult. Because the room could not be changed, the internal reviewer may have scored the instructor higher for doing his best with what was available. The external reviewers were perhaps unable to evaluate the room limitations via a fixed point videotape of the class and scored the instructor lower.

Obviously, there will be limitations to the use of videotape in the preparation of external review materials such as lack of information concerning room environment and a lack of either instructor or student perspective, depending on the position of the camera. The findings of this limited study have motivated the participants to use the project on a larger scale. Limitations include the difficulty of finding external reviewers willing to take the time to complete the evaluation and finding instructors willing to take the time to complete the written and videotape materials in preparation for external review.

Summary

This chapter has applied the nine areas of peer review of teaching discussed by Hutchings (1996) to occupational therapy faculty members to support instructional abilities by using various approaches. These same areas were then used as a template for presentation of the peer review of teaching activities of the IU program. Through similar efforts to promote peer review of teaching, it is hoped that teaching will be elevated to a higher status and both teaching and learning throughout occupational therapy programs will improve. Research efforts must be continued to promote what Boyer (1990) called the "scholarship of teaching" to study what does and does not work beyond the level of individual instructors. ■

References

Barr, R. B., & Tagg, J. (1995, November–December). From teaching to learning: A new paradigm for undergraduate education. *Change,* 13–25.

Bernstein, D. J. (1996). A departmental system for balancing the development and evaluation of college teaching: A commentary on Cavanagh. *Innovative Higher Education, 20*(4), 241–248.

Boyer, E. (1990). *Scholarship reconsidered.* Princeton, NJ: Carnegie Foundation for the Advancement of Teaching.

Davis, J. T., & Swift, L. J. (1995). Teaching portfolios at a research university. *Journal on Excellence in College Teaching, 6*(1), 101–115.

Everly, J. S., Poff, D. W., Lamport, N., Hamant, C., & Alvey, G. (1994). Perceived stressors and coping strategies of occupational therapy students. *American Journal of Occupational Therapy, 48,* 1022–1028.

Hutchings, P. (1995). From idea to prototype: The peer review of teaching: Starting the conversation. *American Association of Higher Education project workbook.* Washington, DC: American Association of Higher Education.

Hutchings, P. (1996). *Making teaching community property: A menu for peer collaboration and peer review.* Washington, DC: American Association of Higher Education.

Malik, D. (1996). External peer review of teaching: A new effort in the chemistry department at IUPUI. In P. Hutchings (Ed.), *Making teaching community property: A menu for peer collaboration and peer review* (pp. 93–96). Washington, DC: American Association of Higher Education.

Seldin, P. (1993). *Successful use of teaching portfolios.* Boston: Anker.

Shulman, L. (1989). Toward a pedagogy of substance. *American Association of Higher Education Bulletin, 8.*

Integrating E-Mail
and the Classroom:
Two Teaching Strategies

Sonia S. Zimmerman

Sonia S. Zimmerman, MA, OTR/L, is Assistant Professor, Occupational Therapy, School of Medicine & Health Sciences, University of North Dakota, Grand Forks, North Dakota.

The technological information age is a dynamic environment that has the power to change our way of knowing and becoming informed as educators and clinicians. Occupational therapy educators are challenged to incorporate technology into already bulging curricula. This chapter describes two ways to bring instructional technology, specifically e-mail, into teaching— one an interactive electronic journal and the other a course listserv. Together, the two assignments are effective to encourage computer use and prepare students for a practice area where knowledge and use of computer technology are increasingly expected. A literature review is provided for each strategy presented as well as advantages and suggestions for the educator considering application.

I T'S EVERYWHERE—TECHNOLOGY, THE INFORMATION AGE, THE information superhighway, cyberspace. References to technology abound. The educational expectations and needs of the 1990s college student are different than those of the past. To prepare students for the ever-changing world of technology, a new paradigm for college instruction is required. Goggin, Finkenberg, and Morrow (1997) suggested that the lecture method alone will be insufficient to meet the needs of these students, and small class teaching methods are often inefficient. Computer-aided instruction offers greater access to instructional assistance during and outside regular class times, individualized pacing, feedback, and collaborative learning. Although new technologies can be overwhelming at times, these technologies have provided educators with increasingly powerful tools to enrich the learning environment (Kizzier, 1995). This article describes two ways to bring instructional technology, specifically e-mail, into teaching.

1. An interactive electronic journal
2. A course listserv

Each assignment has been used in the University of North Dakota's Occupational Therapy Program for a minimum of three semesters.

Strategy 1: Electronic Journals

The major difference between an electronic journal and the traditional course journal is that electronic journal entries are submitted via e-mail, which is mail delivered through electronic means. Student-generated text is transmitted through computers to faculty members for review and comment. Through the journal assignment, the student is asked to reflect on the previous class period, consider his or her participation, include observations of self and others, and provide a record of his or her experience as a group member. In so doing, the student uses self-reflection as a learning tool.

Literature Review

A review of the literature regarding electronic journals across several fields in education yields several relevant studies. Tao and Reinking (1996), in their review of e-mail in education, reported that e-mail communications tend to bring out traditionally silent voices, are motivating and increase interactions between students and instructors, extend the connection of students outside the classroom, and allow students time to reflect before responding, which results in higher-quality responses. Graduate nursing students have reported greater faculty–student communication and more personalized learning as well as a definite increase in computer literacy (Graveley & Fullerton, 1998). McDonnell and Achterberg (1997), in a study of nutrition students, rated the e-mail interaction portion of their distance learning course positively, particularly the timely feedback and time to formulate thoughts and compose messages to the group. Predominant themes in the literature review include increased interaction between students and instructors and more time to reflect and compose thoughts, both of which are useful to the course described.

Application

OT 305: Group Experience is a course designed to promote effective interpersonal communication to prepare the student for professional patient interactions in clinical practice. Emphasis is on the development of basic listening skills, the ability to provide meaningful feedback, sharing personal attitudes and feelings, and appropriate group membership skills. Examples of class topics include self-awareness, values and behavior, effective communication, assertiveness, and dealing with moral dilemmas. Student achievement is measured by participation in class activities, recitation of question responses, and journal entries. In keeping with the knowledge that computer use will be an important practice element of the future, electronic journal entries were chosen as a way to add technology applications to the course. Writing a journal entry provides the student a time and place to reflect on the classroom experience and knowledge exchanged, to pose questions, to see themselves in new ways, and to increase understanding of the importance of the classroom experience to practice (Patton et al.,1997; Tryssenaar, 1995).

Students are assisted in securing e-mail addresses and instructed to use the computers in the university laboratories to submit a weekly journal entry. The basics of using e-mail are demonstrated, back-up handouts are provided, and students who are proficient with e-mail are paired with new learners to learn the technology and ease the transition from keeping a journal to using a computer.

The journals are considered interactive—for each entry the student makes, he or she receives a faculty response via return e-mail and then reads the response before coming back to class. Students comment in course evaluations that the journal entries are a strength in the course: "Journal entries keep us in touch and provide feedback." Informally, students comment, "I have been afraid of computers, but this is fun."

Advantages and Suggestions

The electronic journal has had numerous positive results for both the students and the instructor. Students receive faculty feedback weekly, which encourages ongoing communication between faculty members and students. For example, if there are disagreements among students or common questions regarding the last class period, the instructor knows about it and can bring those ideas or questions to class. With encouragement via instructor response, the students practice their assertiveness skills and bring their own questions to the group, which allows the student to make timely and constructive use of the exchange. Although the learning objective of the journal could be met in traditional paper format, the e-mail journal seems to add novelty and motivation to participate as well as speed of exchange. Additionally, students are introduced to the computer facilities on campus; learn how to be proficient at sending, receiving, and responding to e-mail; and discover other computerized services on campus. The instructor, too, benefits in several ways. Because of the relative informality of e-mail, faculty responses are more likely to take on a conversational quality and often are exchanged more than once before the class period. Strictly from a logistical standpoint, faculty members no longer must collect and carry stacks of journal notebooks (often with hard-to-read handwritten responses) home to correct. All of this is done at the computer with typed student journal responses, and actual response time is often shorter. Suggestions for others who are interested in pursuing this strategy include making sure the students have explicit instruction regarding how to use e-mail and providing adequate access to computers for student use.

Strategy 2: Course Listserv

A listserv provides an opportunity for persons with common interests to communicate via e-mail. This technology allows a person to send a message electronically to one address (the listserv) that will distribute the message to every e-mail address included on the list. A teacher can have a closed list, a course listserv, thus creating a safe environment for class members to continue to interact outside of the classroom. Members of the class can read or send messages whenever it is most convenient for them (Yungbluth & Bertino, 1996).

Literature Review

Powers and Mitchell (1997) reported that, during the listserv discussion, the instructor became less of a knowledge provider, and everyone in the class became part of a community of learners. Kelly (1997), in a study of service learning students required to submit regular e-mail journals, found that students were more aware of their changing ideas and skills and were more connected to their classmates. Wu (1997), in a study of the effects of computer technology on mental process in writing and teaching, reported that students writing about their ideas and choices helps them share memories, fulfillment, and frustrations and facilitates less rule-constrained interchanges where students converse and think together. Yungbluth and Bertino (1996), in a study of an upper-level interpersonal communications class, found participation in the listserv provided social support in learning to use the technology as well as in developing a deeper understanding of the course content. Furthermore, they concluded that, although their study found that those who participated were likely to be the same students who participate in the traditional classroom, the technology served to extend the borders of a classroom community (i.e., provided students an outlet to explore ideas or continue class discussion outside of the classroom). Common ideas include sharing between learners, extending the borders of the classroom, and social support and connectedness as a result of the student's participation in the listserv.

Application

A second application of e-mail involves the use of a listserv in a course entitled OT 304: Psychosocial Aspects of Occupational Therapy With Children, Adolescents, and Young Adults. The course addresses the psychosocial aspects of human development related to the child, adolescent, and young adult. The primary content includes normal psychosocial development, interruptions in development, and mental health occupational theory and practice. Because the content is related to mental health practice and many students have had limited patient contact, class discussion is encouraged throughout the course as a way to identify and dispel stereotypes and myths. However, in a class of 46 students engaging each student is not always feasible. For this reason, the listserv was developed for this course.

Students are invited to subscribe to the listserv and participate in discussion on course topics via e-mail on the listserv. Students who choose this option are earning points for participation in the course, much as they would if they engaged in classroom discussion. Even though it is optional, approximately 80% of the students subscribe each semester, with half of them actively participating and the remainder "lurking" (watching the on-line interaction but not participating). Students' identities are clearly available in the address line of the e-mail.

Early in the course, the instructor poses a question to the students on the listserv for their response. The questions are developed to encourage student learning by integrating course material to practice settings or to challenge the students to think critically about course topics. For example, in the unit on eating disorders, the following questions were posed.

- What are your thoughts about today's guest speaker who shared her personal experience with anorexia and bulimia?
- What would it be like to be her occupational therapist?
- What struggles might you have experienced?
- What concerns do you have for her today in her ongoing recovery?

Later in the course, the following questions were asked.

- How much "individual freedom" do persons with serious mental illnesses really have?
- Does it include allowing people to live on the streets?
- Do others such as mental health professionals, family members, and friends have the right to decide where people should live?

Each of these questions produced a lively discussion with many viewpoints aired.

As the course progresses, students bring the questions to the group and debate them from several angles with little or no instructor facilitation. Students are encouraged to share anecdotes from their own experience (personal, work, or volunteer) and in doing so add a richness to the topic that is appreciated by all. In addition, students, some of whom are otherwise intimidated by large group discussion, have been observed to share their knowledge and provide valuable input to the discussion. For these students, the listserv, where the student is faced only with the computer terminal rather than the faces and nonverbal behavior of his or her classmates, is believed to have the potential to become a stepping stone to increased participation in the traditional classroom.

Advantages and Suggestions

What advantages are there for faculty members? Or is a listserv just more work? Yes, it takes time, but it has been extremely rewarding to witness students engaging in the dialogue of the profession with little or no direct instructor facilitation. It is not unusual to see students who are strong listserv discussants but are silent in the classroom begin to raise their hands in class and participate more by the end of the course. Finally, the course listserv serves as an excellent introduction to the many specialized listservs (American Occupational Therapy Association Special Interest Section listservs, for example) available to both students and professionals. As with the e-mail application described earlier, student understanding of the technology and access to computers is a vital component. Faculty members must be prepared for the ebb and flow of a listserv, which in this case closely followed the students' schedule of examinations and assignments in the occupational therapy curriculum. Encouragement to continue to participate, along with thought-provoking questions, is helpful, as may be additional points granted for responding to a listserv question. Another application of the listserv would be to assist fieldwork students in networking and sharing with each other while in fieldwork and, in doing so, benefit from mutual acquisition of new clinically based knowledge or to similarly connect fieldwork educators with the school's fieldwork coordinator. The possibilities abound.

Conclusion

Observations of course activities support many of the findings of other researchers, specifically extending the borders of the classroom and providing social support with the course listserv. Similar to the findings of Yungbluth and Bertino (1996), many of the strong participants in the course listserv were strong discussants in the classroom. However, there were several instances where students who were otherwise less vocal did begin to voice their ideas and stretch their communication skills. It is believed that the interaction between students and faculty members, at least from the faculty perspective, is much richer with the electronic journals than the traditional journal, which supports the findings of Tao and Reinking (1996). The increased efficiency lends itself well to more frequent dialogue with students, especially those experiencing difficulty. Students report that the electronic journals and listserv activities have increased their overall computer literacy and introduced them to new possibilities (i.e., library searches, the World Wide Web, communication with friends on other campuses).

Together, the two assignments are effective to encourage computer usage and to prepare students for a practice area where knowledge and use of computer technology are increasingly expected. The technological information age is a dynamic environment that has the power to change our way of knowing and becoming informed as clinicians. Occupational therapy education must encourage the development of basic skills for lifelong learning in this age by integrating technology into course work. Already, lifelong learning encompasses much more than reading paper journals, magazines, and attending conferences. It includes participating in listservs, topic searches, downloading full-text articles, on-line conferences, and networking with colleagues in faraway places via the Internet.

Of interest to educators would be further research on instructional technologies, including study of the faculty member–student interaction and what kind of courses benefit most from these strategies, as well as comparing traditional methods with technology approaches. In other words, what are the specific roles that e-mail and listservs play in helping to facilitate learning? Educators are challenged to find ways to use the technology available effectively as tools to improve occupational therapy education and learner outcomes. ■

References

Goggin, N. L., Finkenberg, M. E., & Morrow, J. R. (1997). Instructional technology in higher education teaching. *QUEST, 49*, 280–290.

Graveley, E., & Fullerton, J. T. (1998). Incorporating electronic-based and computer-based strategies: Graduate nursing courses in administration. *Journal of Nursing Education, 37*(4), 186–188.

Kelly, J. (1997, March 12–15). *Effective reflection: Using computer conferencing as the writing component of a service learning course.* Paper presented at the 48th annual meeting of the Conference on College Composition and Communication, Phoenix, AZ.

Kizzier, K. L. (1995). Teaching technology vs. technology as a teaching tool. In N. J. Groneman & K. C. Kaser (Eds.), *Technology in the classroom: National business education yearbook* (No. 33, pp. 10–24). Reston, VA: National Business Education Association.

McDonnel, E., & Achterberg, C. (1997). Development and delivery of a nutrition education course with an electronic mail component. *Society for Nutrition Education, 29*, 210–214.

Patton, J. G., Woods, S. J., Agarenzo, T., Brubaker, C., Metcalf, T., & Sherrer, L. (1997). Enhancing the clinical practicum experience through journal writing. *Journal of Nursing Education, 36*(5), 238–240.

Powers, S. M., & Mitchell, J. (1997, March). *Student perceptions and performance in a virtual classroom environment.* Paper presented at the annual meeting of the American Educational Research Association, Chicago, IL.

Tao, L., & Reinking, D. (1996, October 31–November 3). *What research reveals about E-mail in education.* Paper presented at the 40th annual meeting of the College Reading Association, Charleston, SC.

Tryssenaar, J. (1995). Interactive journals: An educational strategy to promote reflection. *American Journal of Occupational Therapy, 49*, 695–702.

Wu, J. (1997, March 12–15). *Students' conversations we have never heard: Transparencies on the listserv.* Paper presented at the 48th annual meeting of the Conference on College Composition and Communication, Phoenix, AZ.

Yungbluth, S. C., & Bertino, S. (1996, November 23–26). *Extending the borders of community and learning with electronic mail discussion lists.* Paper presented at the 82nd annual meeting of the Speech Communication Association, San Diego, CA.

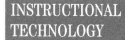
Teaching Occupation-Centered Practice Through Interactive Videoconferencing

Patricia A. Crist

Patricia A. Crist, PhD, OTR/L, FAOTA, is Chair and Professor, Department of Occupational Therapy, Duquesne University, Pittsburgh, Pennsylvania.

This article describes using the full capabilities of interactive videoconferencing equipment to link students in a class on campus with experts on occupation in the profession at their off-campus sites located in Canada and the United States. Staffing two case studies was used to stimulate students' comparative knowledge about different approaches to occupation for interactive discussion with each expert, one at a time. Students interacted with these experts by posing questions and responding to expert queries. The students' final evaluation of this course component that used interactive videoconferencing as an instructional method is reported.

RAPID DEVELOPMENT IN EDUCATIONAL TECHNOLOGY IS CREATING new ways to deliver instruction. For many occupational therapy educational programs, concepts such as the electronic university, distance education, and "the university without walls" are creating innovative methods to deliver occupational therapy curricula. Simultaneously, traditional faculty-centered teaching is being redesigned to focus on student-centered learning approaches (Wingspread Group on Higher Education, 1993). Computer-based instructional technologies such as the Internet, e-mail, on-line discussions (listservs and chat rooms), and quickly emerging "Web-TV" will support new delivery methods such as distance education. Distance teaching or education involves providing learning opportunities to students at remote sites who may be scattered across a wide geographical region, even internationally, without the faculty member's physical presence (Knapper, 1998). With distance education, formal learning is shifted from focus on the faculty expert to focus on the inquiring learner (Plater, 1995). This new focus supports a strategy that can prepare students for lifelong learning.

Academic institutions are developing educational technologies that support the exporting of classes and continuing education to multiple off-campus sites, including satellite campuses, businesses, and directly into the student's home. Academic administration's interest in distance education has emerged to address a "triple challenge."

1. How to live within limited budgets

2. How to make all programs accessible to all students who need them

3. How to help students graduate with the kind of skills, knowledge, and wisdom that they will need to make good starts in the worlds of work, politics, and personal life (Ehrmann, 1995)

Additionally, Ehrmann (1995) stated that the pool of potential learners can consist of all adults because use of distance education technologies eliminates instructional delivery barriers such as classes meeting at prescribed times in prescribed locations, the distance between the learner's community and the campus, access for students with physical challenges, and varying educational preparation and learning styles. Electronic technology creates an open information system and a more flexible model for student–teacher interaction because conventional constraints such as time, place, and use of a common text are no longer essential, and access to information is essential, not supplemental (Plater, 1995). Plater (1995) forewarned that, although the delivery of traditional lectures at distance sites is typically the initial venue, the resources of electronic classrooms are far more vast and limitless.

Distance education knows no real boundaries as exemplified by the western governors' 1996 announcement establishing the Western Governors' University, a regional virtual university that provides interstate delivery of curricula (Leavitt, 1997). Other campuses are rushing to create distance education programs because the marketplace is boundless. As a result, securing quality students will be highly competitive. Comparative analyses of quality, costs, access, and other educational benefits will take on new meaning for both the academy and the learner.

Among occupational therapy educators, the use of distance education strategies is increasingly discussed. Although fascinated with the opportunities for postprofessional education in occupational therapy, skepticism in using distance education is attributed to the need for socialization of professional behaviors and the acquisition of specific skills through typical laboratory activities that are part of entry-level education. Until recently, the use of television to deliver education through video relay to live classrooms was criticized because of a lack of reliable two-way communication access (Knapper, 1998). Now, with instructional system technologists assisting faculty members, the reliability of video and auditory interactive instruction has markedly improved. This video connection provides exciting new approaches to delivering occupational therapy education, including the professional socialization process.

Videoconferencing, one of the numerous approaches to creating electronic classrooms, is rapidly being undertaken by academic institutions to deliver real-time lectures and continuing education. However, the most frequent educational use of interactive video continues to be traditional lecture presentations or faculty-directed discussions through exporting a class to remote student locations. Innovative use of videoconferencing to use the full interactive capabilities of this system for instructional purposes is seldom reported.

Occupational Therapy and Distance Education

The continual quest for excellence in education is built on a traditional teaching foundation but adapted to focus on student learning needs and competence. One major instructional task in occupational therapy education is to teach students how to apply theory to practice. Lecturing and reading about occupation-centered practice is necessary for initial introduction of materials. However, active learning strategies are needed to engage the student in "doing activities" to practice bridging theory and practice. In the past, teaching laboratories have provided the major instructional method for "learn through doing." Recently, methods such as cooperative, case-based and problem-based learning are being implemented in occupational therapy education because they actively simulate students in doing critical thinking and clinical reasoning abilities considered essential to practice.

Now, occupational therapy educators are showing an increased interest in distance education approaches. A survey completed by the Education Department at the American Occupational Therapy Association (AOTA) (Angelo & Zukas, 1997) indicated that 15% of 105 responding programs were currently using distance learning strategies. More important, among the 89 programs not offering distance education, 42 programs (47%) were actively exploring the possibility, with nearly 50% of this group expecting to do so in 2 years or less. Current occupational therapy educational programs offering some form of distance education included 43% for postprofessional education, 22% for associate degrees, and 15% for entry-level students. Survey respondents currently use distance education to deliver traditional educational methods such as lecture (82%) and question and answer (75%) followed by faculty–student discussion (43%) and demonstration (25%). Additionally, the survey indicated that the two most frequently reported concerns were cost and reliability of systems followed by great concern for student's feelings of isolation, lack of active involvement, or interaction with faculty members.

As discussed earlier by Plater (1995), the resources created by the educational technology are far more vast and limitless than currently reported by this AOTA survey. Fuller, more imaginative use of emerging electronic education strategies are warranted in occupational therapy education. Additionally, evaluation of these methods must be undertaken to substantiate claims and identify both strengths and deficiencies in using new educational technologies.

Purpose

The purpose of this report is to describe and evaluate a resourceful use of interactive videoconferencing as an instructional strategy in occupational therapy education. The outcomes from videoconferencing reported here were the result of a major redesign of a capstone course to integrate prior acquired learning into holistic, occupational approaches useful for practice. The class was to be student-centered learning—not faculty teaching-centered learning—to provide students with opportunities to prepare for practice because their Level II fieldwork placements began 2 months after this class. The redesign of this course resulted in two major sections to provide student-centered learning.

1. Interactive video case analysis with experts in occupation approaches to practice

2. Creation of problem-based, tutorial learning groups

The latter process is described elsewhere (Stern, 1998).

The interactive video section of the course reported herein provided students with an opportunity to staff two case studies with individual experts who are developing specific approaches in the use of occupation. The students were linked sequentially with seven experts in occupation approaches through interactive videoconferencing technology, referred to as *V-tel* on our campus. The educational approach was designed to use videoconferencing capabilities effectively, to limit students' feelings of isolation from the learning situation, and for students to actively lead the learning process. Learning was student-centered with the theoretical experts and faculty members serving as consultants during the interactive videoconferences. To use the expert's knowledge efficiently as well as maximize the use of interactive conferencing time to facilitate expert–student interaction, students engaged in traditional educational approaches to prepare for the seminars. This preparation included journal readings, narrative in texts, faculty lecture, and written preparation of case presentations.

Videoconferencing Instruction

The learning process was adapted from the successful interactive learning model presented in *Infusing Occupation Into Practice: Three Approaches* (Crist & Royeen, 1997). In these proceedings, three major theorists in occupational therapy discussed and compared their different approaches with occupational-centered practice by using one common case study (Model of Human Occupation by Dr. Gary Kielhofner, Occupational Adaptation by Dr. Sally Schultz, and Occupational Science by Dr. Florence Clark). As a result, learners (in this case, the conferees) were able to compare the clinical relevance and advantages of each of the approaches with each other. An unexpected insight for both the conferees and, now, readers is understanding how each theorist developed their approach to occupation by reflecting their past experience and environmental context for practice integrated with their professional values and individual personality.

By using videoconferencing capabilities, this workshop experience was adapted for classroom application by having students staff the same two case studies in the presence of each individual major theorist separately. As a result of the active engagement in the case-learning method with the expert, the students' learning would be reinforced regarding each theory. The interactive video sessions included: Ecology of Human Performance (Dr. Winnie Dunn), The Model of Human Occupation (Dr. Chris Helfrich), Occupational Adaptation (Dr. Janette Schkade), Occupational Science (Dr. Florence Clark), Person–

Environment–Occupation (Dr. Mary Law), Person–Environment–Performance (Dr. Carolyn Baum), and Spirituality (Dr. Chuck Christiansen).

Implementation of Interactive Videoconferencing Instruction

All students were given the same two case studies adapted from Dunn, Brown, McClain, and Westman (1994) (a child with learning disabilities in school and a man who had a stroke) and subdivided into teams of four students for each theory or approach. One dyad would staff the pediatric case and the other dyad would staff the adult case through videoconferencing with each expert while the class listened. Separate videoconferencing links were established between the campus site at Duquesne University (Pittsburgh, PA) with university campuses in Texas, Kansas, Illinois, California, Missouri, and Canada.

Before the videoconferencing session, students wrote their responses to the objectives for the staffing of their case: What are the main performance problems? What would you evaluate? Where would you begin treatment? What would be your anticipated occupational outcomes? What were problems you had in applying this specific approach? Reflective study of class readings and lectures coupled with self-initiated consultation with campus faculty members contributed to the students' written preparation for their interactive video-conference session.

At an established time, all students gathered in the two-way, interactive videoconferencing classroom on campus to do the presentations of case studies and for the class to talk with the expert. Each 1.5- to 2-hr session included a brief overview by the expert, followed by a separate presentation of each case by the assigned student dyads, and then general discussion by all participants. Students were required to use the language and characteristics of their assigned approach to occupation during staffing. The electronic technology permitted real-time discussion and visual interaction between the expert and students. The session was concluded by the expert identifying current strategies and research they were engaging in to further develop their approach to occupation. Each session was videotaped.

Outcomes from V-Tel Sessions on Occupation

Because this was the first time this student-centered course was delivered in this format, extensive student feedback was solicited. Oral and written, formative and summative, and formal and informal sources were gathered to monitor learning, student satisfaction, and course adaptation. The summative, written evaluation of the students was extensive and covered all aspects of the course. Only the course outcomes related to the V-Tel application are reported here.

The quantitative student feedback of the V-tel experience is reported in Table 1. Before this course, 20 of the 22 students reported no prior experience with videoconferencing technology, with 2 students saying they had three previous experiences. Student evaluations indicate overall positive results in the videoconferencing interaction with the occupational therapy experts at the conclusion of the course.

Session Content

Overall, students agreed that they acquired new learning from these sessions. In evaluation narratives, several students requested that more lectures on each

Table 1
Averaged Results of Interactive Videoconferencing Course Evaluation

Evaluation of Videoconferencing Session Content	
1=strongly disagree, 2=disagree, 3=no opinion, 4=agree, 5=strongly agree	
1. V-tel sessions were interesting.	4.0
2. V-tel sessions facilitated my understanding of each approach to occupation.	3.9
3. V-tel sessions improved my professional communication skills.	3.9
4. V-tel sessions were appropriate to my level of knowledge and skill.	4.1
5. V-tel sessions helped me with clinical problem solving.	3.7
6. The use of V-tel interaction with experts in occupational therapy is valuable.	4.4
Evaluation of Videoconferencing Session Technology	
1=terrible, 2=poor, 3=fair, 4=good, 5=excellent	
1. Sophistication level regarding knowledge of us and technology.	3.4
2. Quality of in-class video projection.	4.1
3. Quality of in-class audio projection.	4.3
4. Switching of cameras from instructor to audience.	4.2
5. Ability to see students when they talked.	4.2
6. Ability to hear persons from other sites.	4.2
7. Quality of handouts or projected visual aids from instructor.	3.4
8. Interactive video provides a learning experience that is just as effective as live instruction.	4.0
Overall course evaluation including video sessions (list of relevant items only)	
1=strongly disagree, 2=disagree, 3=no opinion, 4=agree, 5=strongly agree	
1. Exploration of current ethical dilemmas as they occur in health care delivery.	4.4
2. Overall, I have more confidence in my treatment planning skills.	3.6
3. Overall, I feel better prepared for fieldwork.	3.8

Note. N = 22 students.

approach to occupation be given before V-Tel sessions and that lectures on an approach be followed immediately by the same session. Certainly scheduling busy experts in different time zones when equipment at both ends was available was a challenge that could be corrected with coordination beginning no later than 6 months before the session.

Students indicated moderately improved communication skills, understanding of approaches to occupation, and development of clinical problem solving through the use of video technology. These lower ratings could be the result of

- an insufficient amount of faculty lecture to synthesize information prior to session,

- self-reported limited ability of the problem-based learning instructors to clearly apply the approaches to occupation during problem-based learning sessions that were to reinforce student knowledge and application, and

- only requiring the four students assigned to present during the V-tel session to do preparatory writing of their presentation, which leaves other students to be passive recipients and not be actively engaged or accountable for each session.

Consequently, some students were not able to discriminate approaches, as indicated by the following comments. ·

- "Although thoughts, ideas, and theories in occupational therapy can be different, they all seem to result in the same outcome in the end."

- "Preparing me for fieldwork, exposing me to models but at the same time confusing me because there were so many models."

However, a larger group of students saw the unfolding differences and unique contributions each approach to occupation made to practice applications. For instance, one student noted:

> I also feel that I have a good understanding of the different theories for practice in OT, and I have a feeling of true importance of carrying this theoretical knowledge with me when I practice…I think that the most valuable learning experience was actually getting to talk to the theorists and hearing their perspectives…how their theories fit into OT.

Secondary benefits included students being exposed to the potential of new learning technology as well as having the opportunity to practice professional communication approaches with noted experts in occupational therapy. Additionally, students better understood the motivation for the expert's approach and how the interaction between an expert's philosophy and the practice environment results in the development of a unique approach to occupation.

Interestingly, several students provided unsolicited feedback after Level II fieldwork. They praised the V-tel learning opportunity after they had experienced practice, stated that more activities similar to this one needed to be included before fieldwork, and indicated that many of their fieldwork educators were envious of this learning opportunity. Although this was pleasing to hear, the future course needed to engage all students in student-facilitated discussions or learning activities, not just dyads, to further synthesize, compare, and contrast the different approaches to occupation.

Student Motivation for Learning

Whenever a class is delivered, multiple instructional approaches are used to promote learning. This class was clearly designed for student-centered learning and was noted by students as more desirable than traditional methods. Interestingly, the quantitative ratings as well as the individual qualitative statement demonstrated the students' motivation for active engagement. As discussed previously, the intentional use of only two case studies during V-Tel was to allow comparison between the approaches by having the case studies remain unchanged so that learning was focused on the approach to occupation and not the uniqueness of each case study. However, a few students believed that repetitive use of the two cases was limiting their preparation for practice and was even boring.

Students noted how this active learning instructional strategy motivated and enhanced their knowledge and skills.

- "When I participate more, I learn more."
- "I think it helped me think through cases more effectively."
- "I learned more about resources, my own clinical reasoning and ability to form treatment plans."
- "I definitely saw an increase in the amount I learned. I was not as bored, and my attention was better."

Regarding the actual interactions with experts, feedback included the following comment:

> I think I spent more time preparing for V-Tel because I knew I was speaking to the developer of the theory gave me confidence when speaking. It made me an active participant in my own learning process, making myself more responsible for my own acquisition of knowledge.

Clearly, the use of videoconferencing stresses students' active and interactive capabilities and reinforced acquiring new lifelong learning abilities more than just content acquisition.

Session Technology

The technology was evaluated by the students as reliable. This is attributed to the quality of the system and, most important, the preplanning and presence during all sessions of the campus videoconferencing technologist. All links with sites were piloted by the technologists from each site several days before class, and all links were established 30 min before the class began. The results from items 1, 7, and 8 used to evaluate the videoconferencing session technology necessitate further reflection.

■ Item 1: Although students gained a solid respect for this technology, this lower rating may have occurred because they were recipients of watching the system in operation and not actually running it themselves.

■ Item 7: Because this was the first time more experts used V-Tel in this manner, much was learned about how to prepare these materials for projection. Whenever linking sites, no matter how sophisticated our campus system was, the quality of the system is reduced to the lowest audio and visual projection quality available. As a result, some of the audio and visual transmissions were not of similar high quality, and some were even distracting.

■ Item 8: Although the overall high rating demonstrates students regard for interactive video, three students strongly disagreed that the use of V-Tel was as effective as live instruction. This finding warrants future attention to evaluate if this resulted from frustration with new technology, change in typical instruction modes, or some other reason.

Overall Student Course Evaluation

In general, students reported that this course prepared them for practice expectations. In comparing the three major instructional approaches, problem-based learning in small tutorial groups was most valued followed by the interactive video sessions. Faculty-centered lecture was evaluated as the least relevant for future practice. This hierarchy reflects the degree of student- versus faculty-centered instruction discussed earlier. The problem-based learning sessions were seen as far more pragmatic, but several students wrote that the V-Tel clearly assisted them in articulating the relationship between theory and practice. Because Level II fieldwork began soon after this course, student anxiety regarding their ability to perform was nearly peaked by the time this class ended and the summative data was gathered. Because this class ended just before fieldwork, the lower ratings for confidence and fieldwork preparations may reflect confounding issues for these two items. Several members of the class did report pre-fieldwork anxieties through these clinically relevant challenges during the video sessions.

Interestingly, students noted how the interaction between the expert and their current practice contexts resulted in understanding the personality behind their approach to occupation and how their background and interests guided development of their approach to occupation. This resulted in students' enhanced perspectives of the approach and the experts and their skills as developing students. Sixteen students supported this outcome through similar writing exemplified by the following comments in response to V-Tel activities.

■ "Interaction with the people who developed and used these frames of reference on a daily basis. It was interesting to see how and why their views developed."

■ "I understand things better when someone explains them to me, and these were the people who designed the theories, so they were the best to explain."

■ "We were able to gain a better understanding by interacting rather than simply reading."

■ "The interaction with other professionals who were interested in how we approached a case and what we had to say."

The primary use of videoconferencing to help students increase their knowledge about approaches to occupation by using interactive contact with experts was substantiated in this course. This result may indicate the positive possibilities of developing increased curriculum content delivery through expert faculty members from distant locations.

Student Professional Development and Skills for Lifelong Learning

Professional socialization outcomes such as the following were evident.

■ "The opportunity to interact with someone other than faculty, to present myself and my ideas in a professional manner and to have a chance to talk to a few highly regarded OTs."

■ "Learning how to interact with another professional in a more confident and assertive manner."

■ "Had a chance to learn and apply a frame of reference to a case and have immediate feedback and discussion."

Costs for Delivery

Costs for using the V-Tel technology to import nonuniversity faculty members included telephone-line time for the campus telecommunication, links with the site from our end, a uniform honorarium to the experts, and any additional costs related to linking to systems at the site of the experts. This cost to link outside systems was highly variant. Sometimes, system use was free if being used by faculty members for instructional purposes. Other times, a minimal access charge and fees for the experts' on-site technologist were charged. Still, the costs were far lower than bringing the expert in for a seminar. In one case, a school's charges for connection far exceeded the typical costs charged for videoconferencing equipment usage. A cheaper rate was located at a nationwide commercial copying center. When we requested that the expert link through this public entity to reduce costs, she relayed this desire to her technologist who adjusted their fee to be comparable to this business.

Closing Comments

Two unanticipated outcomes will result from this experience because all sessions were simultaneously videotaped with the permission of the experts. Faculty members and several adjunct faculty members had used the tapes for their own professional development. The background materials along with observing the tape have become in-service materials for faculty members. Second, the experts were curious about the outcome comparisons between approaches because all used the same two cases. As a result, qualitative content analysis of the transcribed video sessions is now underway to uncover similarities and differences in each approach to occupation in general as well as specifically for each case study.

Whenever an instructional technology or approach is implemented in a classroom, faculty members should know its effectiveness and plan evaluation of the process as it unfolds. Likewise, campuses and accreditation processes must support faculty members risking the use of new instructional techniques and not penalize them for doing thoughtful risk taking during annual review or tenure processes. Even experienced lecture faculty members must reengineer their course content to make relevant use of videoconferencing capabilities and maximize student learning. All occupational faculty members should embrace study of their educational practices because "Our Practice is Education!" (the motto of the 1995–1998 Education Special Interest Section Standing Committee).

Student-centered, interactive videoconferencing with experts in the profession appears to have great potential for the future of occupational therapy education. To simply use these systems to deliver lectures at distance sites does not use the full potential of the system. Likewise, although the interest in exporting education to remote sites accelerates, similar benefits for importing education may be as profound for the educational preparation of our future occupational therapy practitioners, not to mention providing stimulating professional development seminars. Potential intercampus bartering agreements for exchanging faculty expertise between campuses could be less costly while markedly improving the quality of education. ■

Acknowledgment

Tracy Saur collaborated with the author in the actual delivery of this course, which used V-Tel technology for the first time. Her organizational ability is acknowledged. Likewise Boris Valic, our interactive video technologist from Duquesne University (Pittsburgh, PA), was indispensable in planning and implementing the video links between sites.

References

Angelo, J., & Zukas, R. (1997, April). *Reaching beyond the classroom: New methods of teaching at the professional level.* Paper presented at the annual conference of the American Occupational Therapy Association, Orlando, FL.

Crist, P. A., & Royeen, C. B. (Eds.). (1997). *Infusing occupation into practice: Three approaches*. Bethesda, MD: American Occupational Therapy Association.

Dunn, W., Brown, C., McClain, L. H., & Westman, K. (1994). *The ecology of human ecology: A contextual perspective on human occupation.* Bethesda, MD: American Occupational Therapy Association.

Ehrmann, S. C. (1995). Introduction. In E. Boschmann (Ed.), *The electronic classroom* (pp. i–iv). Medford, NJ: Learned Information.

Knapper, C. K. (1998). Technology and college teaching. In R. E. Young & I. E. Eble (Eds.), *College teaching and learning: Preparing for new commitments* (pp. 31–46). San Francisco: Jossey-Bass.

Leavitt, M. O. (1997). A learning enterprise for the cybercentury: The Western Governors University. In D. G. Oblinger & S. C. Rush (Eds.), *The learning revolution: The challenge of information technology in the academy* (pp. 180–194). Boston: Anker.

Plater, W. M. (1995). In search of the electronic classroom. In E. Boschmann (Ed.), *The electronic classroom* (pp. 3–13). Medford, NJ: Learned Information.

Stern, P. (1998). Skills for teaching: A problem-based learning faculty development project. *American Journal of Occupational Therapy, 52,* 230–233.

Wingspread Group on Higher Education. (1993). *An American imperative: Higher expectation for higher education*. Racine, WI: The Johnson Foundation.

Examination of Fieldwork Educators' Responses to Challenging Situations

Ruth S. Farber

Kristie P. Koenig

Ruth S. Farber, MSW, PhD, OTR/L, is Assistant Professor, and Kristie P. Koenig, MS, OTR/L, is Assistant Professor, Department of Occupational Therapy, College of Allied Health Professions, Temple University, Philadelphia, Pennsylvania. This research was supported by the Dean's Incentive Fund of the College of Allied Health Professionals, Temple University, Philadelphia, Pennsylvania.

Background: *Fieldwork education is facilitated through the supervisory relationship. As in all human relationships, conflicts or problems may emerge. It is important to know how current occupational therapy fieldwork educators approach and mitigate these challenges, especially in light of fieldwork setting shortages.*

Objective: *The purpose of this exploratory study was to examine the types and range of supervisory strategies used by fieldwork educators and to examine their thinking about strategy implementation—particularly when problematic situations occurred.*

Method: *Data was collected from an initial focus group and follow-up group and telephone interviews. Qualitative methodology for data analysis was used with the constant comparison method of grounded theory.*

Results: *A taxonomy of interventions was developed to prevent or respond to challenging fieldwork situations. The main approaches used by fieldwork educators were student-centered, supervisor-centered, or supervisory structure-changing interventions. A supervisory reasoning process emerged that reflected the fieldwork educators' perceptions of the students' behavior and educators' thoughts about choice, timing, and use of appropriate strategies.*

T HE FIELDWORK EXPERIENCE IS AN INTEGRAL PART OF THE educational and professional development of occupational therapy students. It is facilitated primarily through the supervisory relationship (Christie, Joyce, & Moeller, 1985a). Simultaneously, the supervisory experience has meaning to fieldwork educators and is an important part of their professional development (Griswold & Strassler, 1991). Student–supervisor relationships are often enriching and gratifying; however, as with all interpersonal relationships, conflict and strain may occur (Farber, 1998; Kanazawa, 1990). This may seriously affect the quality of the experience and cause stress for both members of this relationship (Farber, 1998). In addition, the fear of a problematic situation may deter clinicians from becoming fieldwork educators (Tompson & Proctor, 1990) or prevent practicing fieldwork educators from taking on additional students. This situation is particularly salient in light of the existing shortage of fieldwork sites, which has been described as a "national crisis" (Cohn & Crist, 1995).

The shortage of fieldwork sites and the need for more fieldwork educators is compounded by the lack of uniform preparation and training for fieldwork educators (Christie, Joyce, & Moeller, 1985b; Cohn & Frum, 1988; Crist, 1996; Opacich, 1995; Vestal & Seidner, 1992). Although there has been progress in the development of resources for fieldwork training to remove it from its neglected status (Cohn & Crist, 1995, p. 103), continued refinement and development of both theoretical and practical supervisory training resources unique to contemporary occupational therapy practice are important. Resources for training fieldwork educators can be enriched by information regarding the handling of challenging fieldwork situations that are specific to current occupational therapy fieldwork education practices.

Challenging Fieldwork Situations

When a challenging situation occurs in fieldwork, it is important to consider the systemic perspective including the supervisor, the supervisee, their interaction, and the setting (Loganbill, Hardy, & Delworth, 1982). In surveying fieldwork supervisors, Christie et al. (1985b) inquired about the primary problems confronting them. These fieldwork educators identified students' "attitudinal and affective behaviors" (Christie et al., 1985b, p. 678), including lack of interest, as a major problem and lack of supervisory problem-solving skills. The need for fieldwork educators to develop more effective feedback skills was frequently mentioned, including "difficulty providing negative feedback and confronting students" (Christie et al., 1985b, p. 679). Kramer and Stern (1995) used a case study method to describe some types of problems that can occur in fieldwork. They found that students who had difficulty engaging actively in supervision and taking responsibility for their own behavior, as well as difficulty receiving and responding to feedback, had problems with fieldwork supervision. Farber and Weiss (1997) found that the behaviors mentioned above were problematic for fieldwork educators and that this was due to the perception that these situations required extra time and energy and increased stress (Farber, 1998). Within the larger, fast-moving climate of managed care in which there is increased accountability for time, the need for additional supervisory resources may be perceived as problematic due to scarcity of time to adequately resolve the situation.

Supervisory Interventions

Occupational therapy practitioners are highly resourceful people who are skilled at facilitating adaptations, creative problem solving, and helping people overcome obstacles. These abilities could be applied to challenging fieldwork situations as well. Frum and Opacich (1987) have contributed to knowledge formation of supervisory resources through the application of conceptual principles from the seminal, developmentally based model of supervision by Loganbill et al. (1982). This model examines and describes a range of supervisory interventions as well as other aspects of supervision. Regarding supervisory interventions, Loganbill et al. (1982) described the possibilities involved:

> The total pool of intervention strategies available to the supervisor is rich, varied and like the total possible moves in a chess game, infinite in number. Some of these interventions can be described as skills and specific techniques and some may be described as more nurturing conditions or environments which the supervisor may set up. These may include attitudes and philosophies which prevail but are difficult to pinpoint into discrete definable interventions. (p. 3)

Although relevant and applicable to occupational therapy, Loganbill and associates' (1982) model was originally developed from supervisory interventions used in the field of counseling psychology. To develop the occupational therapy training literature, it would be important to examine the supervisory interventions that reflect practice within this field. Moreover, with the increased complexity of practice, the continued need for preparation of fieldwork educators and the changing health care system, empirical exploration of the nature of relational problem-solving in this field would be useful. Therefore, the purpose of this study is twofold.

1. To understand and categorize the repertoire of intervention strategies used to prevent or respond to problematic behavior

2. To explore the thinking of fieldwork educators about use of intervention strategies for particular situations

Methodology

Background

In a prior study, our research focus shifted from the problematic behavior of students to the fieldwork educators' comfort with specific interventions and the general types of strategies used (Farber, 1998; Farber & Weiss, 1997). This earlier study contained an exploratory question to uncover general types of responses that fieldwork educators found helpful to deal with problematic behavior. The responses fell into two general categories.

1. Student-focused strategies such as opening communication, clarifying expectations, or increasing structure

2. Supervisor-focused strategies such as seeking support from colleagues or the academic fieldwork coordinator

These categories guided and stimulated our thinking in approaching the current study. To expand and explore these preliminary findings, it was believed that further research was needed to examine the fieldwork educators' responses in depth and to examine the way they implemented their response choice. The focus group format (Kreuger, 1994) provided an opportunity to obtain descriptive information about perceptions and thoughts regarding this process.

A focus group of fieldwork supervisors ($N = 8$) was conducted. Two researchers were present in the focus group. Before the group began, it was decided that one researcher (a faculty member from the previous study) would conduct the group interview and facilitate discussion. The other researcher, the current fieldwork coordinator, observed and recorded nonverbal interaction and noted speakers' contributions for accuracy of transcription. The main questions asked were

■ What is problematic in terms of student behavior (for you)?

■ How does this type of student behavior affect you?

■ What strategies have you used, and how did they work?

To obtain a range of perspectives, participants from various settings and with various degrees of experience were invited. Out of 11 invited, 8 agreed to attend (the other 3 were not available for scheduling reasons). Of the participants, 2 worked in psychiatric settings, 5 worked in physical disability or rehabilitation settings, and 1 worked in a pediatrics setting. They were all women, and their collective years of experience as occupational therapy practitioners ranged from 3 to 15 years ($M = 7$). Their years of experience as fieldwork educators ranged from 2 to 9 years ($M = 5.2$).

After the group meeting, the researchers met for a debriefing session (Kreuger, 1998). Data were analyzed and summarized and sent to all members of the focus group. For data verification, member checks (Cresswell, 1994) were conducted. A second follow-up focus group ($n = 2$) was conducted for this purpose as well as for further exploration of this topic, followed by a debriefing between the investigators. Because it was difficult for some fieldwork educators to attend the second group, 3 respondents were interviewed by telephone for the same purpose. These contacts lasted from 30 to 60 min. The total respondents followed up ($n = 5$) included group and telephone interviews. Questions asked of all 5 respondents were

■ Overall, do the findings reflect your experience of the supervisory process?

■ Are there any clarifications or additions?

In addition, some questions were asked about the timing and sequencing of the strategies they used.

Data Analysis

Within the qualitative paradigm, data collection, analysis, and interpretation occur concurrently (Cresswell, 1994). The audiotapes of the focus groups and debriefings were transcribed to ensure data completeness. Then both researchers individually reviewed the transcripts, made provisional codes in the margins of the transcript, and when possible used in vivo coding (i.e., the participants' own words) (Strauss, 1987; Strauss & Corbin, 1990). New data were compared and contrasted with previous data by using the constant comparison method of grounded theory (Strauss & Corbin, 1990). Through subsequent discussions, second focus groups, and analysis and reanalysis of the data, the researchers' individual codes were synthesized into larger categories. A taxonomy of the central interventions used by the fieldwork educators was formed. This process included a review of strategies generated from the previous study (Farber, 1998). Kreuger (1994) advocated the use of triangulation of focus group data with other types of data sources "to confirm findings and to obtain both breadth and depth of information" (p. 30). It was found that the responses from the previous study could be subsumed and confirmed under the new categories and subcategories developed. In addition, themes that transcended specific strategies emerged and were noted.

Findings

The final taxonomy developed contained the range and types of fieldwork intervention strategies used to prevent or react to problematic behaviors (see Tables 1–3). The terms *interventions* and *strategies* seem to be used somewhat interchangeably in the literature (Frum & Opacich, 1987). For the purpose of this study, the term *interventions* will be reserved for the three broad-based categories that indicate the direction of the activity, whereas the specific subcategories will be referred to as *strategies* because they are specifically action based. The three main categories that emerged in the current study were

1. student-centered interventions (including proactive, reactive, and active problem solving; reflective strategies; and the facilitation of support),
2. supervisor-centered interventions (including proactive, active, and reflective strategies and seeking support), and
3. supervisory structure-changing interventions (including changing the supervisory ratio, clinical setting, and actual supervisor).

There was a diversity of response and variety of sequences regarding the handling of challenging student situations. Fieldwork educators sometimes sought supervisor-centered interventions such as feedback from their colleagues and then approached the student more comfortably and constructively. Other times, this process worked in reverse with the fieldwork educator consulting a colleague after an unsuccessful or puzzling interchange with a student. Structural changes such as a change in supervisors occurred usually after the student- or supervisor-focused strategies failed.

The relationship between problematic behavior and supervisor strategy was not a simple one and appeared to be mediated by many factors. These factors included the type of student behavior, the supervisor's conception (internal representation) of the problem and accompanying sense of urgency to respond, the supervisor's expectations of students at a particular point in the fieldwork

Table 1
Student-Centered Interventions

Proactive (student orientation and preparation)

- Clearly state expectations and responsibilities of student (sometimes in writing)
- Facilitate activities that orient student to staff members
- Review safety and infection control checklist with student

Reactive (immediate or timely direct action)

- Identify and directly approach student about problematic behavior
- Address safety or hygiene concerns immediately or as soon as possible
- Address student for being judgmental toward patients or staff members
- Set direct expectations for time-sensitive written records

Active problem solving

- Set up a contract (with specific goals, behaviors, or learning objectives) and timeline
- Use a mid-term evaluation by the student to clarify expectations and concerns
- Maintain, improve, and open communication (in general or with specific techniques)
- Increase general feedback as well as positive feedback to build self-esteem and effectiveness
- Use active strategies to foster student competence (role playing or group problem solving)
- Plan physical unavailability (when safe) for students who hold back

Reflective

- Understand cause
- Get more information and discuss issues with the student; seek the student's solutions
- Suggest self-monitoring (student sets weekly goals and reports back informally)
- Build empathetic understanding of the patient
- Facilitating student supports
- Provide student groups for support and problem solving
- Pair with a person from another discipline
- Call a faculty member or FWC as a student advocate
- Promote a "village" orientation and opportunity for multiple learning experiences

process, the supervisor's approach to problem solving, the experience level of the supervisor, and the organizational context. Because the data from this study was voluminous (as is often the case in qualitative studies), the researchers decided to report on two of the themes that influenced the orchestration of strategy use.

Table 2
Supervisor-Centered Interventions

Proactive

■ Develop Level II fieldwork supervisory preceptorship, supervisory orientation, and training

■ Supervise Level I students before Level II (balance types of students)

Active problem solving

■ Gather information (observe the student in other situations with other staff members)

■ Learn different communication strategies and change the style of feedback

Reflective

■ Self-examination or self-monitoring (Am I modeling what I am asking student to do?)

■ Depersonalize behavior and feedback (not intentional)

■ Readjust expectations (this person is a student)

■ Learn from experience and adjust behavior for the next student

Seeking support

■ Get feedback regarding perceptions from colleagues

■ Call or arrange meeting with academic fieldwork coordinator for collaboration or support

■ Develop a collaborative training network, versus sole responsibility, for the student

1. The importance of timing

2. Willingness to change the course (initial behavior was not what it seemed)

Importance of Timing

The importance of timing of the supervisor's response was mentioned in different ways ranging from the importance of "clearing the air" before the (relationship) problem had gone too far or correcting problematic behavior before it happened again or became worse. Two specific areas in which timeliness of supervisory response was particularly salient for the group members were safety and infection control issues and "unprofessional" appearance and demeanor.

Safety and infection control issues: "So much at stake." Safety issues included safe transferring, proper hygiene procedures, and medical vulnerabilities of patients (e.g., swallowing precautions, need for cardiopulmonary resuscitation). With the safety issues, the fieldwork educator first tried to prevent damage by using student-centered proactive strategies (orientation of the student) and reactive strategies (to respond quickly). For instance, if a patient is about to fall, or a student goes into the bathroom without gloves, the supervisor

Table 3
Supervisory Structure-Changing Interventions

Change the ratio of supervision

■ Pair more and less experienced supervisors to clarify expectations

■ Bring in an additional supervisor (co-supervise)

■ Bring in additional students (for peer support)

■ Increase structure or provide additional informal supervision

■ Change clinical settings (improve the goodness of fit)

■ Transfer the student to a clinical setting with a different pace of practice

■ Change supervisors

■ Use for entrenched personality conflict (after other approaches are tried thoroughly but unsuccessfully)

either addressed the issue immediately with the student or took the student aside soon after. A fieldwork educator mentioned infection control and emergency procedures. She described what she tells students.

> Make sure you're washing your hands. Glove up before you take them in the bathroom. You know, constant reinforcement, because maybe they've not ever been in a hospital setting where they have to be concerned about it. I always go over the infection control and safety department plans like I would for a new employee…so it makes me not forget to tell them where the…bag is for CPR and what is the difference between a stat and a code… It's a ready-made checklist for me, and that way I'm sure I've done it.

There is much thought about student sensitivity, as well as maintaining the image of the hospital, when there is a potential safety risk. The fieldwork educator continued in a way that demonstrated her concern for the multiple parties involved.

> Well, we don't want the patients to think the staff or the students are incompetent. You don't want the student to feel bad when they're trying to do something…But yeah, right after the transfer [problem], I stick them in the office and say I think that maybe next time you should consider these things…Thanks for trying.

This fieldwork educator and others in the focus group implemented this type of (student-centered) reactive strategy, which emphasized a didactic and immediate approach to teaching the appropriate steps and procedures required for safety. In contrast, the following fieldwork educator's perception of addressing safety issues as part of a larger normative process occurring over time allowed her to use reflective strategies.

> Students will have safety questions. It happens to all of us when we had to handle an incident. Because accidents happen. Some students may get caught up in

their own thought process in terms of what they are doing and what their treatment is. They may need some reminders of the consequence. Did you consider that this could be a safety risk? It is the first time that the patient has been up ambulating, and are you having them do a complex meal task? Sometimes I think the student gets caught up in the treatment planning and great ideas with what to do with the patient and forgets about some of the other safety issues. I think that is an ongoing process. I think that is a developing process, too. When the students first start working with a patient, they are working in the box and not really taking in the whole picture. That comes with experience.

This supervisor explained that she does a lot of questioning to foster student (and employee) awareness of the effect of their behavior on others in the system.

"Unprofessional" appearance and demeanor. Professional appearance and demeanor seemed important to several supervisors. Supervisors were concerned about the image of the profession ("my profession") as well as the image of the hospital. Because appearance issues like gum chewing, untied shoelaces, and so forth were brought up as problematic behaviors, the fieldwork educators were asked how they respond. One fieldwork educator described her belief in the necessity of an immediate response by using a (student-centered) reactive strategy regarding gum chewing.

I attack that right head on—from day one, an hour later, you know what I mean? Do you think it looks nice if you're walking down the hall chewing gum? Be realistic. And I try to just say, take a look at yourself in the mirror and talking to a patient and it just doesn't really look nice so...No, no, things like that, I don't want them coming in tomorrow, just with something very basic, you know...I mean, certainly with a patient issue or other things like that I—we— have weekly meetings regardless. But things that are very basic like that, I correct. And I would never do it [correct] in front of the patient, never make the student feel like you know, they're this big, but I pull them aside in a quiet environment.

In contrast, another supervisor saw the issue of unprofessional appearance differently, and therefore the timing of response was not as critical an issue.

I'd respond in a timely way, although my perception of dress may not be the same as someone else's. For example, if someone came with open-toe shoes, it is a safety issue and against policy. Or a low-cut top, it could create a problem of interaction with patients. If it doesn't go against any rules, I may talk about it, but not in a timely way. I wonder if personal preference is an issue for some people. We have a loose standard here. We can wear jeans that are not blue or faded...In some ways, our dress code can be considered loose and unprofessional. (On some units there is more hands-on work.) Rehab has more body fluids. Some units dress up a bit....If they are in the office and they are doing something like chewing gum, I'm fine with it. I set the limits before they start. I guess it falls under being proactive. Within the office, you can be more loose, can talk freely. Once you're outside the store, you are portraying professionalism to the

> rest of the department and other standards hold true. Look at the unit and see how they function and see them as role models.

In contrasting the approaches mentioned in the quotations from the two previous fieldwork educators, the latter demonstrates the educator embedding the perception of the problem within a larger context and showing organization and subtleties of thought and approach (as well as incorporating reflective and proactive strategies). Unexpectedly, this was found to parallel some aspects of the clinical reasoning process. (This type of unexpected finding can emerge in qualitative analyses.) Robertson (1996) suggested that the first part of the reasoning process includes the understanding of the problem (or the person's internal representation of the problem). Robertson (1996) found that experienced clinicians (in comparison with students) had elaborate "well developed schemata" that allows them to tap into a larger "network of information" (p. 213). This could contribute to an expansion in accompanying interventions and problem-solving processes. It is possible that more experienced supervisors show these more advanced thinking qualities or that some supervisors use more complex schemata either because of personal characteristics (i.e., cognitive flexibility, psychological sophistication) or type of supervisory experience or training.

Willingness To Change Course: Initial Behavior Was Not What It Seemed

A fieldwork educator described the following scenario in which she had an initial perception that changed with time and further reflection. Subsequently, the fieldwork educator was willing to change the course of her behavior with a student who had been at her facility for 1 week.

> I first thought she was blowing things off. I thought I needed to take immediate action and confronted her [reactive strategy]. I basically gave her an ultimatum to think...about making a decision...is this the setting for you?....It was Friday and I told her to think about it over the weekend.

The supervisor subsequently thought about it as well (supervisor-focused, reflective strategy) and was worried about being too quick to react or hurting her potentially supportive role. The supervisor realized that the pressures she was under influenced her sense of urgency. In a subsequent discussion that was more mutually reflective, she discovered what she originally perceived as unconcern was actually that the student felt paralyzed. The student was not used to the expectations of this setting or the population and had personal issues that became "stirred up."

Similarly, another fieldwork educator demonstrated her willingness to change strategies as well as the process that unfolded as she tried to understand her student's initial "obscure" behavior.

> A female student who was trying hard. She didn't look like she was organizing things right, she looked inept, and she didn't look like she knew how to interact

with patients, but her paperwork was very good [laugh]…And the behavior was obscure to me. I didn't know what the problem was. She wasn't being a competent beginning new affiliate student….And…if I couldn't figure out what was going on…she would be at risk for failing the affiliation….I couldn't help her. She was new at this. She can't tell me the problem….She was so bad in one area and good in the other….So I meet with her periodically for a couple of weeks, trying to get more information from her on individual things, like her running groups. Initially I gave her more concrete suggestions [active problem-solving]…kinda helped at first. This is what you do, this is the timeline.

Then I called up the FWC [fieldwork coordinator], relatively early. I was at such a loss at what to do. My normal strategies were not working. The FWC confirmed that the student is academically able to do things….With the FWC, I brainstormed [supervisor-centered, seeking support, and active problem solving] other ways to handle it and…gave other strategies that I hadn't thought of….In discussion something helped me click things together. We talked about developmental learning….She said some students learn gradually, and for some students it all comes together at once….It put it together for me. The student is trying to do things at a high level of learning….Also the FWC talked about the student liking theory, learning and doing things perfectly…it gave me a different way of handling it again.

When I talked to the student again. I said "You seem very interested in the patient. You are trying so, so hard. You seem very interested in theory and trying to be accurate"…That helped open up a different way for the student to give me information [reflective strategy]. So the student started to talk about trying to apply all these theories….And she was trying to be precise, getting all the information accurately, and feeling responsible for what if this person should go home and do something wrong.

Because I reframed my questions, she was able to talk to me a little bit different. And it came together more….The student was an overly responsible individual…and was trying to apply theory and working to remember and incorporate them. I said "I like that, but you need the fundamentals." Then I made an analogy of…trying to ride a bicycle (like a high-speed racing bike) in traffic, up a hill, and doing everything at once. Whereas right now I just need you to ride in a straight line, on a flat surface, with no traffic, no people, nothing around. That is the timeliness, that is the basic structure. I don't want you to worry about all the theory right now, I just want you to focus on this self-care element and getting the groups timely in the next week. Once you get comfortable with that, then you can add some complexity to that. That analogy worked for her.

This above example demonstrates how the interaction with the FWC (seeking support) facilitated the fieldwork educator's own problem solving, which in turn enabled her to interact with her supervisee successfully. This sequence demonstrates how supervisors may go from student-centered active problem-solving interventions to supervisor-centered seeking support and then go back to rework learning interaction with student-centered strategies.

Supervisory Reasoning

As mentioned earlier, parallels of the supervisor's reasoning process and the clinical reasoning process emerged again while analyzing the data. We chose to describe the reasoning process of supervisors they observed as *supervisory reasoning*. In the situation described above, the fieldwork educator's reasoning appears similar to what Fleming (1991) described as *continuous reasoning*, which entails "a continuous stream of small decisions or temporary hypotheses" (p. 992). "Experienced therapists seemed to be constantly revising their plans, not because they did not get it right the first time, but rather to fine tune the plans in accordance with the patients' needs, wishes, body, abilities and limitations" (Fleming, 1991, p. 992). In the situation described above, the supervisor's responsiveness and individualization of approach appeared to facilitate the development of the supervisee as well.

Discussion and Implications

This study delineated and categorized a repertoire of strategies occupational therapy fieldwork educators used to prevent or mitigate challenging situations and examined their approach to different strategies. In this research, a *supervisory reasoning* process emerged that appeared to parallel various aspects of the occupational therapy practitioners' clinical reasoning process and affected the timing and approach to use of problem-solving strategies. Although results of qualitative studies such as this one are not generalizable, the ample descriptions can be useful as a practical resource for fieldwork educators, as a resource for training of fieldwork educators, and as a guide for future research.

For both the fieldwork educator and student, the interpersonal supervisory environment has been found to distinguish good from poor fieldwork experiences (Christie et al.,1985a). Because there are challenging times in all human relationships, awareness of increased possibilities for creative problem solving is fundamental to the strengthening or rebuilding of the training relationship if conflict occurs. It is interesting that many of the specific student-focused interventions are similar to those embedded in Christie et al.'s (1985a) findings of the description of critical components of a good fieldwork experience, including quality and timeliness of feedback and communication as well as the clarity of learning objectives. The action that the fieldwork educator takes to prevent or mitigate problems may be part of the normative foundation of good supervisory practice.

It is important for the fieldwork educator to be cognizant of how and when they optimally intervene with students. For some fieldwork educators, giving immediate feedback (i.e., correcting clearly inappropriate dress, underscoring safety rules) seemed to "clear the air," establish the rules, and allow them to go on with the supervisory process. In a previous exploratory study (Farber, 1998;

Farber & Weiss, 1997), it was found that fieldwork educators who were more comfortable with prescriptive interventions (i.e., giving a definite plan of action for a specific situation) were less likely to see problematic behavior as serious. There are times when students need practical limits. In contrast, there are other situations, such as when behavior is more ambiguous or the result of strong underlying affect (such as anxiety), where a more reflective and unfolding approach would be preferable. Knowing how and when to respond to the student to be most effective is part of the art of supervision. This is not clear, especially for the novice. The decision-making process that fieldwork educators used to make these choices appeared to be guided by a reasoning process described in this chapter as *supervisory reasoning*.

The supervisory reasoning process reflected the fieldwork educators' perceptions of the students' behavior and their thoughts and appropriate action. Like the clinical reasoning process, the supervisory reasoning process showed variation in the way supervisors understood the students' behavior (internal representation of the problem) (Robertson, 1996), students' ability to generate hypotheses and entertain competing hypotheses (Fleming, 1991), and how supervisors made ongoing changes to individualize their approach with students (continuous reasoning) (Fleming, 1991). Although several participants with more years of supervisory experience displayed increased complexity in this supervisory reasoning process and approach to problem solving, experience itself was not uniformly associated with this kind of thinking in all participants. In addition to experience, other factors that may influence the development of supervisory reasoning, such as the practice context and training in supervision, need further exploration.

Special training and orientation to become a fieldwork educator were described as helpful by several of the respondents. Several fieldwork educators described how calling the academic FWC became easier with experience. It seems to be essential for fieldwork educators to feel safe asking for help (supervisory-focused interventions) not only for challenging situations but also to share ongoing fieldwork education responsibility. Therefore, the development of sources for training and support (i.e., American Occupational Therapy Association regional fieldwork consultants or fieldwork consortia and mentoring networks) is essential.

Last, because this was an exploratory study, further research of this subject is recommended with a larger sample. Further validation and elaboration of the intervention strategies and implementation is encouraged. Additional exploration of supervisory reasoning is suggested, including the examination of the factors that influence the development of supervisory reasoning, the relationship between the complexity of the reasoning of the fieldwork educator and the development of clinical reasoning in the student, and differences between novice and expert supervisors. ▪

Acknowledgments

Special thanks to Donna Weiss, PhD, OTR/L, FAOTA for her thoughtful involvement in earlier aspects of this research.

This article is partially written on the basis of preliminary data from a paper at the American Occupational Therapy Association's 1998 Annual Conference and Exposition, Baltimore, MD ("Occupational Therapy Supervisors' Solutions to Fieldwork Dilemmas" and is briefly mentioned in the *Education Special Interest Section Quarterly* (Farber, 1998).

References

Christie, B. A., Joyce, P. C., & Moeller, P. L. (1985a). Fieldwork experience. Part I: Impact on practice preference. *American Journal of Occupational Therapy, 39*, 671–674.

Christie, B. A., Joyce, P. C., & Moeller, P. L. (1985b). Fieldwork experience. Part II: The supervisor's dilemma. *American Journal of Occupational Therapy, 39*, 675–681.

Cohn, E. S., & Crist, P. (1995). Nationally Speaking—Back to the future: New approaches to fieldwork education. *American Journal of Occupational Therapy, 49*, 103–106.

Cohn, E., & Frum, D. (1988). Fieldwork supervision: More education is warranted. *American Journal of Occupational Therapy, 42*, 325–327.

Cresswell, J. W. (1994). *Research design: Qualitative and quantitative approaches.* Thousand Oaks, CA: Sage.

Crist, P. A. (1986). *Contemporary issues in clinical education.* Thorofare, NJ: Slack.

Farber, R. S. (1998). Supervisory relationships: Snags, stress, and solutions. *Education Special Interest Section Quarterly, 8*(1), 2–3.

Farber, R. S., & Weiss, D. (1997, April). *Perceptions of problematic fieldwork behaviors and supervisory intervention.* Paper presented at the annual conference of the American Occupational Therapy Association, Orlando, FL.

Fleming, M. H. (1991). Clinical reasoning in medicine compared with clinical reasoning in occupational therapy. *American Journal of Occupational Therapy, 45*, 988–996.

Frum, D., & Opacich, K. J. (1987). *Supervision: Development of therapeutic competence.* Bethesda, MD: American Occupational Therapy Association.

Griswold, L. A., & Strassler, B. (1991). Formulating a fieldwork philosophy and resources. In E. B. Crepeau & T. LaGarde (Eds.), *Self-paced instruction for clinical education and supervision (SPICES)* (pp. 21–39). Bethesda, MD: American Occupational Therapy Association.

Kanazawa, Y. (1990). *Management of conflict in psychotherapy supervision.* Unpublished doctoral dissertation, Temple University, Philadelphia, PA.

Kramer, P., & Stern, K. (1995). Case Report—Approaches to improving student performance on fieldwork. *American Journal of Occupational Therapy, 49*, 156–159.

Kreuger, R. A. (1994). *Focus groups: A practical guide for applied research.* Thousand Oaks, CA: Sage.

Kreuger, R. A. (1998). *Analyzing and reporting focus group results*. Thousand Oaks, CA: Sage.

Loganbill, C., Hardy, E., & Delworth, U. (1982). Supervision: A conceptual model. *The Counseling Psychologist, 10*(1), 3–42.

Opacich, K. J. (1995). The Issue Is—Is an educational philosophy missing from the fieldwork solution? *American Journal of Occupational Therapy, 49*, 160–164.

Robertson, L. J. (1996). Clinical reasoning. Part 2: Novice/expert differences. *British Journal of Occupational Therapy, 59*(5), 212–232.

Strauss, A. (1987). *Qualitative analysis for social scientists*. New York: Cambridge University Press.

Strauss, A., & Corbin, J. (1990). *Basics of qualitative research: Grounded theory procedures and techniques*. London: Sage.

Tompson, M., & Proctor, L. F. (1990). Factors affecting a clinician's decision to provide fieldwork education to students. *Canadian Journal of Occupational Therapy, 57*(4), 216–222.

Vestal, J., & Seidner, K. (1992). The clinician as student educator: Coaching vs educating. *Occupational Therapy Practice, 3*, 29–38.

A Model of Fieldwork Consortium Development

Kristie P. Koenig

Caryn Johnson

Kelly McCarron

Kristie P. Koenig, MS, OTR/L, is Assistant Professor and Fieldwork Coordinator, Department of Occupational Therapy, Temple University, Philadelphia, Pennsylvania.

Caryn R. Johnson, MS, OTR/L, FAOTA, is Fieldwork Coordinator and Instructor, Department of Occupational Therapy, Thomas Jefferson University, Philadelphia, Pennsylvania.

Kelly A. McCarron, MEd, OTR/L, is Instructor, Duquesne University, Department of Occupational Therapy, Rangos School of Health Sciences, Pittsburgh, Pennsylvania.

Portions of this article were presented at the state conference of the Pennsylvania Occupational Therapy Association, October 1997, Pittsburgh, Pennsylvania.

Fieldwork education is the vital link between the classroom and the clinic. Currently, educational institutions and clinical communities are faced with a turbulent health care environment, dwindling resources, and expanding student populations. The "crisis" in fieldwork is a reality for academic fieldwork coordinators, fieldwork educators, and students. Organizational efforts to provide quality fieldwork education are all-encompassing. Interinstitutional collaboration is a viable, efficient option to increase joint efforts on the local, state, and national levels. This article provides a model for interinstitutional collaboration—the consortium. The developmental process of the consortium is emphasized to provide a structure that encourages collaboration at all stages. Survey results from both new and established consortia are shared to illustrate the variety and uniqueness of organizations that desire collaboration. Key elements for consortium functioning are identified to enhance performance and productivity.

"**F**ACING THE FIELDWORK CHALLENGE" IS A CATCH PHRASE IN occupational therapy literature, a reality among academic and fieldwork educators, and a growing concern to an increasing student population. As occupational therapy and occupational therapy assistant programs are expanding and developing, the effects of managed care are affecting the ease with which fieldwork sites can commit to Level I and Level II students. Necessity has resulted in the development of innovative fieldwork models, group supervision, and nontraditional placements that have had a positive influence in changing the face of fieldwork education. These market-driven changes have opened doors to new practice areas, provided peer support for students in collaborative models, and extended services in traditional and community settings. Academic fieldwork coordinators (AFCs), fieldwork educators (FWEs), and students have been at the core of these changes, working together to elevate fieldwork education and build bridges between the classroom and practice. A vehicle that has supported this development is the fieldwork consortium. The purpose of this article is to provide a description of a model of fieldwork consortium development with case examples generated from various fieldwork consortia throughout the country.

The development of fieldwork consortia in the United States is limited, but six leaders in the fieldwork consortia community provide an illustration of the different collaborations in the country at this time. The Appendix illustrates the different stages of development for each of these consortia. Some are in their infancy, whereas others appear advanced in the developmental scheme outlined.

Although a consortium-based approach to fieldwork is not a new concept, institutions are now, more than ever, faced with the need to collaborate to meet the charge to educate future practitioners. Structurally, individual states, schools, or regions may create a unified body for the purpose of fieldwork education (e.g., Wiscouncil, which serves Wisonsin, and the New England Occupational Therapy Education Council). Smaller metropolitan areas with many programs have chosen to form collaborative groups to be more effective with their fieldwork programs and pool resources to benefit all members involved. Regardless of the structure, collaboration is the key to success in today's fieldwork climate.

The proposed model of consortium development is not intended to be a fixed template but rather should be viewed as a fluid example of the potential to collaborate when unity is desired. The individual educational programs will reap the benefits of collegial relationships and interdependence. More important, if collaboration is modeled, the clinical community will support endeavors that are no longer viewed as "competitive efforts." If fieldwork coordinators find themselves in competition with their counterparts for limited resources, the potential for burnout is high, and stress becomes an inevitable occurrence. By examining the elements that surround the development of a fieldwork consortium, occupational therapy educators can begin to see not only the process but also the possibilities for collaboration.

Literature Review

To conceptualize consortium development, a discussion of the purpose and reasons that institutions choose to collaborate is necessary. There is a dearth of information in the occupational therapy literature about development and use of fieldwork consortia, although there are published efforts about the outcomes of consortia activity (Brown, Caruso Streeter, Stoffel, & McPherson, 1989). Much of the literature on use and development of consortia can be found in nursing with its historical movement of educational programs out of hospitals and into university settings (Styles, 1984; Walker, 1985). This movement created a rift between nursing education and nursing service (Walker, 1985) and increased the need for collaboration. Developmental issues related to the use of consortia and collaborative groups in health care have been identified. Styles (1984) formulated a conceptual model of unity that ranged from no communication at one end of the spectrum to complete unification at the opposite extreme. However, in the middle, is where she identified the trend to collaborate. These areas included successively stronger models of communication, consultation, consent, and unified policy, with joint projects being a natural extension of this collaboration. These concepts are the heart of consortia activity.

Humphreys (1996) noted that consortia may differ in exact structure, but the key is effective performance. The performance of consortia will be high if members set aside organizational self-interest for the greater benefit of collective action. In addition, members must see a benefit to justify their participation, have administrative support, and view the relationship as a vehicle to meet their identified needs (Humphreys, 1996; Walker, 1985). Once the decision is made to work together, effective interaction results when members share common interests. A fundamental compatibility and a strong commitment to a clear purpose are likewise beneficial. Members have a willingness to accept responsibility for helping each other (Dufault, Bartlett, Dagrosa, & Joseph, 1992; Earp, Capka, Davis, McLain, Ney, & Moorhead, 1992; Walker, 1985). Barriers to effective collaboration include competition, "turf" issues, fear of losing autonomy, mistrust, mechanics of coordination, time, and funding issues (McPartland, 1991). Earp and associates (1992) discussed how trust must be developed to form a positive, supportive mechanism to achieve organizational goals. McPartland (1991) identified the consortia as a resource and catalyst to foster excellence. Common themes emerge from the discussion on consortium development that address affective, organizational, and professional development components.

The Consortium Model

A model for consortium development in the realm of occupational therapy fieldwork education was developed by the authors to both illustrate how consortia evolve and to provide direction for consortia that want to develop further (Figure 1). Three domains that compose the model have been identified.

1. Affective domain
2. Organizational domain
3. Professional development domain

Each domain has three equally important components that develop concurrently. Each component includes three stages (early, middle, and later), which are organized developmentally. Corresponding Tables 1 through 3 include the developmental stages of each component as well as activities that correspond with each stage of development. Although this is not an all-inclusive list, these activities may generate ideas for other consortia in various stages of development. Some consortia may choose to limit collaboration to a basic level by planning and participating together in activities such as fieldwork educator training workshops and clinical council days. Others may opt for more in-depth involvement by sharing databases and mailings to the clinical community and pooling resources. One should not necessarily infer that greater collaboration is better; rather, collaboration may occur successfully at various stages, and individual consortia determine the level of collaboration that works best for them (Humphreys, 1996).

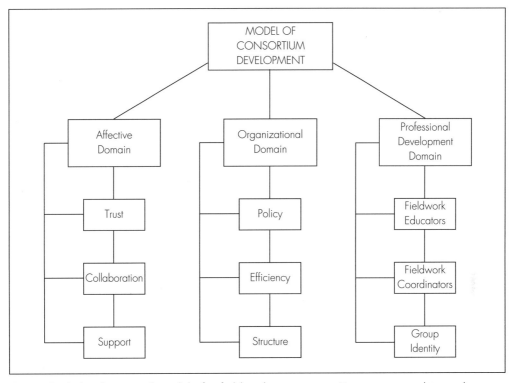

Figure 1. A developmental model of a fieldwork consortium. Components within each domain have developmental stages.

Affective Domain

The affective domain consists of three parallel components.

1. Trust
2. Collaboration
3. Support

Within each of these components, developmental stages exist. Because these components relate to issues arising from the interpersonal realm, they have been termed *affective*. This domain provides the contextual foundation for interactions between members. Because trust, collaboration, and support are inherent to the functioning of a consortium, development in this domain must occur for a consortium to develop in the organizational and professional domains (Dufault et al., 1992; Earp et al., 1992) (see Table 1).

Trust

Today's health care environment and the growing number of occupational therapy and occupational therapy assistant educational programs have contributed to

Table 1
Affective Domain

Domain	Developmental Stages	Developmental Activities
Trust	1. Interaction	■ Meetings of core group members ■ Sharing general information and field-work experiences ■ Commiseration ■ Planning
	2. Mutual accountability	■ Ability to rely on others to carry their own weight
	3. Trust	■ Share more sensitive information such as unused fieldwork reservations, fieldwork database
Collaboration	1. Mutual interests	■ Collaborate on increasing the number of fieldwork sites ■ Discuss methods for handling students having difficulty with fieldwork
	2. Shared goals	■ Invest efforts in collaboration with others ■ Share responsibilities equally among core members
	3. Integration	■ Create a vision ■ Philosophical agreement ■ Members are recognized by community as collaborators rather than competitors
Support	1. Need for support	■ Commiseration ■ Share methods for handling students having difficulty with fieldwork
	2. Validation	■ Discuss various strategies and outcomes ■ Try each other's strategies
	3. Strength	■ Function as resource for others

the current fieldwork crisis. Increasing numbers of students and a finite number of fieldwork sites set the stage for a competitive environment in which schools in close proximity find themselves vying for the same limited number of fieldwork sites. Schools with long-standing programs and well-established relationships with fieldwork sites may resent having to share those sites with the "new school on the block," especially if that means losing valuable reservation spots to the new program. This may be the hardest barrier to overcome in consortium development. As educational programs learn to rely on each other, demonstrate

Table 2
Organizational Domain

Domain	Developmental Stages	Developmental Activities
Policy	1. Compare and contrast programs 2. Adapt and accommodate 3. Policy Development	■ Discuss various policies used by schools and sites within consortium ■ Implement aspects of policies developed by others that are more effective ■ Consider affecting policy on national level (e.g., create resolutions for AOTA regarding fieldwork)
Efficiency	1. Simplify tasks 2. Combine duties 3. Redefine roles	■ Use same format for fieldwork reservation forms ■ Develop universal Level I evaluation form to be used by all schools in consortium ■ Joint sponsorship of fieldwork workshops ■ Share database ■ Joint mailings ■ Universal reservation forms ■ Identify project leaders
Structure	1. Informal 2. Responsibilities emerge	■ Collaboration between fieldwork educators and fieldwork coordinators regarding issues ■ Generate inclusion criteria for members ■ Elect officers ■ Obtain funding from schools, grants, sponsors, etc.

Note. AOTA = American Occupational Therapy Association.

accountability, experience increased support, and begin to be more comfortable sharing, trust will develop.

Collaboration

The whole is greater than the sum of its parts. Consortium members must subscribe to the belief that there is value in working together. The degree to which consortia decide to collaborate will vary widely. As the consortium develops, members share increasingly in the benefits such as increased communication with the fieldwork community, an increased number of fieldwork sites, and heightened efficiency with reservations and programming, and begin to envision mutual goals. The group norm shifts from competition to collaboration.

Table 3
Professional Development Domain

Domain	Developmental Stages	Developmental Activities
Fieldwork educators	1. Training and support	▪ Provide support and materials to local fieldwork educators ▪ Continuing education (training workshops, clinical council days) ▪ Use of competence self-evaluation ▪ Recognition, thanks, awards
	2. Develop expertise	▪ Incorporating local fieldwork educators into the educational process ▪ Assist with development of fieldwork educational materials (publishing and presenting)
	3. Research and development	▪ Research ▪ Evaluate current models and develop new ones ▪ Disseminate information by way of publication and presentation at local, state, and national levels ▪ Assume positions in state and national occupational therapy organizations
Academic fieldwork coordinators	1. Basic management	▪ Establish new fieldwork sites ▪ Train students and fieldwork educators ▪ Manage student placements
	2. Broaden scope	▪ Disseminate information by way of publication and presentation at local, state, and national level
	3. Research and development	▪ Research ▪ Evaluate current models and develop new ones ▪ Disseminate information by way of publication and presentation at local, state, and national levels ▪ Assume positions in state and national occupational therapy organizations

Table 3 *(cont.)*

Domain	Developmental Stages	Developmental Activities
Group identity	1. Local effect	■ Consortium meetings
		■ Provide minutes
	2. Expanding effect	■ Communicate at state and local levels (e.g., newsletter)
	3. Broad effect	■ Participate in national AOTA, Commission on Education

Note. AOTA = American Occupational Therapy Association.

Support

The need for support from others in similar roles is probably the reason most consortia develop in the first place. As that basic need is met, one becomes more competent (and confident) in one's role as FWE or AFC, experiences personal growth, and draws strength from the experience of collaborating.

Organizational Domain

The organizational domain addresses the operation and management of fieldwork-related business and the functioning of the consortium. Development in this area moves from informal to formal structure, and from focusing efforts at the local level to expanding influence and effect to a broader, perhaps national, level (see Table 2).

Policy Development

Every academic program and fieldwork site establishes policies regarding fieldwork education. Policies address issues such as supervision, length of Level I fieldwork experiences, student assignments, types of settings required for fieldwork experiences, and methods for evaluating student performance. When FWEs and AFCs share information with each other about their policies, they often see components of policies used by others that may work well in their own settings.

Efficiency

One of the most helpful contributions a consortium can make to the clinical community is to simplify fieldwork management whenever possible. Another contribution is to provide training to local FWEs. Initial activities to increase efficiency such as joint sponsorship of FWE training workshops, require minimal trust and risk taking, yet yield major benefits to those involved. More advanced activities, such as sharing a database like Fieldwork Clerk (Dudley & Ward, 1996–1998) require higher levels of trust but eliminate duplication of effort. Heightened efficiency decreases demands on FWEs and AFCs alike. Ultimately, consortia may choose to identify nonoverlapping roles for members and identify project leaders on the basis of individual strengths and interests. For example, the AFC from one school may take responsibility for organizing FWE training workshops, whereas the AFC from another school may be responsible for maintaining the database.

Structure

As the structure of the consortium develops, it becomes more complex and more formal. Initially, the group may meet informally, and member roles and responsibilities are similar and equal. Decision making is usually by consensus, and membership structure is fairly open. As the consortium develops, members may find value in a more formalized structure that more clearly delineates roles and responsibilities, determines membership criteria, and defines a governing body. More sophisticated activities often require financial support, and various ways of obtaining funding can be explored.

Professional Development Domain

This domain focuses on the professional development of consortium members (FWEs and AFCs) and on the developing maturity of the group itself. As members' skill and expertise increase, they may engage in more advanced activities such as publishing, presenting, and research and model development, with experienced members mentoring less experienced members. The consortia may consider expanding their focus from local to national as the group matures (see Table 3).

FWE Development

New FWEs begin developing skills in the areas of basic student and fieldwork management and advance to mentoring or training other FWEs. Academic FWEs who are often skilled in publishing and presenting can provide support to less experienced practitioners who are interested in this type of professional development. This developmental hierarchy parallels performance areas outlined in the occupational therapy roles document (American Occupational Therapy Association [AOTA], 1993) from entry-level to high-proficiency skills. The consortium can give structure and support to assist the FWE in setting and obtaining goals as an educator.

AFC Development

At the entry-level stage, AFCs are concerned with the basics of fieldwork management (AOTA, 1993). Management continues, but the AFC may now seek to provide training opportunities to enhance fieldwork educators' knowledge and skills (AOTA, 1993). As their academic careers grow, they are likely to pursue opportunities to publish and present. Experienced AFCs may be motivated to conduct research on the different fieldwork models they use and on various aspects of student performance. They may become interested in developing new fieldwork models, such as group supervision and off-site supervision models, in conjunction with interested FWEs.

Group Identity

The fieldwork consortium is likely to be highly visible in the occupational therapy community because of the need for AFCs to communicate with scores of occupational therapy practitioners on a frequent basis. Publicizing the collaborative efforts of the consortium will generate growing support and interest. Highly productive consortia disseminate valuable information and are looked to for knowledge and leadership.

Conclusion

Ginzburg (1981), a health policy economist, stated "…every occupational group…recognizes that, as a precondition for advancing the well-being of its members, it must organize itself" (p. 28). By organizing into an effective collaborative model, the group will gain influence and have some control over its destiny (Walker, 1985). The "occupational group" committed to fieldwork education can use the consortium model to develop a purpose, foster interaction, provide support, meet organizational goals, bridge AFC and FWE concerns, contribute to practice, and advance models of fieldwork education. Trust, risk taking, and patience are required. However, the eventual benefits easily override the potential barriers.

The developmental consortium model is a tool that AFCs and FWEs can use to review the performance of an existing consortium, open up dialogue and mentoring on current effective consortia, and offer guidance to newly developing groups or those that simply have a desire to collaborate but do not know where to begin. Consortia structure will vary, but by recognizing the need to build and strengthen relationships between institutions, the function and purpose for excellence in fieldwork education will remain central. The potential for consortia to bring about qualitative and effective change in fieldwork education and professional development of its members is considerable. ■

Appendix

Fieldwork Consortia Survey Results

How was your fieldwork consortium originally formed?

Consortium 1   Fieldwork coordinators from three local schools met in Seattle at the American Occupational Therapy Association conference and discussed combining their efforts for a local clinical day.

Consortium 2   Virginia Commonwealth University was the only school in Virginia and formed the Richmond area fieldwork council with local fieldwork clinicians. This council expanded as more schools developed.

Consortium 3   Our consortium started more informally approximately 10 years ago by approximately 4 occupational therapy fieldwork coordinators in our city. At that time it was more of a "coffee clutch" and offered support to people.

Consortium 4   Approximately 15 years ago it started as a group to resolve fieldwork issues relative to our area. It served to educate and assist clinical supervisors.

Consortium 5   Our consortium started 2 years ago to maintain unity in the area occupational therapy programs, to coordinate fieldwork schedules, to revise and use a Level I assessment, and to assist clinical supervisors.

Consortium 6   Several years ago our COE group expanded and formed a local consortium to include all interested academic programs in the Midwest.

How many academic programs are currently involved?

Consortium 1   Five.

Consortium 2   Four occupational therapists and four occupational therapy assistants.

Consortium 3   Academic fieldwork coordinators from 14 occupational therapy and occupational therapy assistant programs along with four clinical representatives from the areas of mental health, geriatrics, physical disabilities, and pediatrics.

Consortium 4   Twenty-five.

Consortium 5   Three.

Consortium 6   Three professional programs, two technical programs, and one associate technical program. We are in the process of adding two professional and one more technical program.

Is there inclusion criteria to become a member?

Consortium 1   No specific member fee. Membership can get support from the university as needed (e.g., $100). There must be a collaborative effort to expand fieldwork sites.

Consortium 2   No.

Consortium 3   Programs must have a developing status from the Accreditation Council for Occupational Therapy Education or be accredited.

Consortium 4   No criteria. Open to all academic and clinical coordinators and supervisors throughout New England.

Consortium 5   No criteria.

Consortium 6   Primary criteria is a fully accredited status, but a few other criteria exist as well.

Where are the meetings held and how often?

Consortium 1   One time per month at local restaurants.

Consortium 2   Meetings are held four times per year in rotating clinical sites.

Consortium 3   Meetings are held in New York City on a monthly basis except for the months of July and August.

Consortium 4   Meetings are held from September to May in mid- to southern-New England on a monthly basis.

Consortium 5   Meetings are held at one location on a monthly basis from September to May.

Consortium 6   Meetings are held at one location on a monthly basis with telephone conference options for distant programs.

Do you have outside sponsorship on which you rely?

Consortium 1   For our bigger clinical council events, we receive support from local agencies. For bigger projects, we receive funds from local district POTA.

Consortium 2   No. Speakers volunteer, the clinical site provides refreshments, and the university sends out all mailings.

Consortium 3   No. Funds for activities are raised by an annual job fair.

Consortium 4   No. Only membership dues.

Consortium 5   No.

Consortium 6   No. We charge a nominal fee for an annual workshop. There is a fee charged for an occupational therapist/occupational therapy assistant exam review annually. We fundraise by selling items with our logo attached.

What types of activities take place at the meetings? Is there a regular agenda? What types of activities do consortium members collaborate on?

Consortium 1   Agenda changes on the basis of the needs of members, but typically we have program updates, peer support discussions, plan for upcoming presentations, and development of collaborative projects (i.e., database, universal reservation form, universal Level I evaluation).

Consortium 2   We have an agenda that includes an update from all schools present and a program related to fieldwork. We include time for networking.

Consortium 3   Yes, we do have a regular agenda. We formed task forces this past year to work on specific projects that worked quite well. We send out our Level II reservation requests on the same date.

Consortium 4   Yes, regular agendas involve discussion regarding relevant fieldwork issues, planning regarding which regional workshops to financially assist, and planning consortium-sponsored workshops.

Consortium 5   The agenda varies due to the newness of the group.

Consortium 6   The monthly agenda is determined by the steering committee chair. We plan spring and fall workshops, discuss promotion of our consortium, discuss ways to serve the membership, collaborate on fieldwork scheduling, and work collaboratively on the revision of our mission and standards.

Do you have a voting body? Who is responsible for making the decisions?

Consortium1   The voting process is done on the basis of a consensual decision reached by the five representatives from the academic fieldwork programs. We encourage input and advice from our four clinical members.

Consortium 2   The leader in our group works closely with the co-chairs. Voting for the co-chairs, secretary, and others is accomplished by including all members present at the meetings.

Consortium 3   A formal structure was imposed this year. A chairperson and secretary were elected due to the growing size of membership. Each member in the group has one vote.

Consortium 4   Yes, there is a voting body consisting of the "steering committee," which consists of an academic representative from each school and one corresponding clinical representative.

Consortium 5   No, we are a new consortium, therefore, there is no need at present.

Consortium 6   Yes, we have a steering committee consisting of a chair, a chair-elect, a secretary, a treasurer, and a nomination chairperson. All of these positions are elected clinical fieldwork supervisors from the general membership. We have one fieldwork representative from each academic program.

Is there a definite mission or bylaws?

Consortium 1   No, we have developed a mission statement but do not have formal bylaws.

Consortium 2   Yes, we have a standard operating procedure.

Consortium 3   Yes, we have bylaws.

Consortium 4   Yes, there is a mission to support the academic and clinical aspects of occupational therapy education.

Consortium 5   No, we are just starting our consortium.

Consortium 6   Yes, they are currently in revision.

Acknowledgments

The authors gratefully acknowledge representatives from various consortia across the country who completed the survey and provided us with insightful case examples. We additionally thank Donna Weiss, PhD, OTR/L, FAOTA, and Kathy Swenson Miller, MS, OTR/L, for their efforts in interinstitutional cooperation that "showed us the way."

References

American Occupational Therapy Association. (1993). Occupational therapy roles. *American Journal of Occupational Therapy, 47*, 1087–1099.

Brown, S., Caruso Streeter, L. A., Stoffel, V. C., & McPherson, J. J. (1989). Development of a Level I evaluation. *American Journal of Occupational Therapy, 43*, 677–682.

Dudley, S. G., & Ward, D. E. (1996–1998). Fieldwork clerk [Computer software]. Ft. Lauderdale, FL: Healthwealth International.

Dufault, M. A., Bartlett, B., Dagrosa, C., & Joseph, D. (1992). A statewide consortium initiative to establish an undergraduate clinical internship program. *Journal of Professional Nursing, 8*, 239–244.

Earp, J. K., Capka, M. B., Davis, A. E., McLain, R. M., Ney, C. A., & Moorhead, J. J. (1992). Enhancing quality critical care education: Establishing a consortium. *Journal of Continuing Education in Nursing, 23*, 15–19.

Ginzburg, E. (1981). The economics of health care and the future of nursing. *Journal of Nursing Administration, 11*, 28–32.

Humphreys, J. (1996). Education commissioning by consortia: Some theoretical and practical issues relating to qualitative aspects of British nurse education. *Journal of Advanced Nursing, 24*, 1288–1299.

McPartland, P. A. (1991). Consortium development: A mechanism for delivering health education programs. *Health Values, 15*, 30–39.

Styles, M. M. (1984). Reflections on collaboration and unification. *Image: The Journal of Nursing Scholarship, 16*, 21–23.

Walker, D. D. (1985). Nursing education and service: The payoffs of partnership. *Nursing and Healthcare, 6*, 189–191.

Exploring Student Perceptions of the Part-Time Therapist/ Full-Time Student Placement

Ann M. Bossers

Mark Hartley

Ann M. Bossers, BScOT, MEd, OT(C), is Associate Professor and Fieldwork Coordinator, and Mark Hartley, Hons.BA, is Research Assistant, School of Occupational Therapy, The University of Western Ontario, Elborn College, London, Ontario, Canada.

The pilot projects that form the basis of the information presented in this study were initiated by the Ontario Council of University Programs in Rehabilitation Sciences through a grant from the Ministry of Health of Ontario, Canada. Previous presentation of material contained in this article is from a paper titled *The part-time therapist/full-time student fieldwork placement* (Bossers, Desrosiers, Jung, Anthony, & Gage, 1997/June). This paper was presented at the Canadian Association of Occupational Therapists conference, Halifax, Nova Scotia, Canada.

Fieldwork placements typically occur in a 1:1 student:practitioner model. In a province-wide study in Canada, 14 occupational therapy students of different levels were matched with a part-time (10 to 30 hr/week) fieldwork educator to complete full-time block placements. These placements are referred to as the part-time therapist/full-time student (PTT/FTS) fieldwork model. The themes that emerged through qualitative analysis of journals completed by student participants in PTT/FTS placements delineate numerous positive features of the model. This article discusses the student perceptions of this model; and outlines the themes, roles, and responsibilities of part-time practitioners who educate students in full-time placements; and the educational value of several learning strategies that are integral to the PTT/FTS model.

R APID CHANGE IS ALTERING THE WAY HEALTH CARE IS PROVIDED in North America (Stanton, 1997). Although an understanding of the full effect of this change must await future consideration, two facts are clear.

1. Rehabilitation has expanded from institutional settings such as hospitals into community settings such as private practice, residential care, education, and industry.

2. Health care resources are being greatly reduced by an economically driven restructuring of the health care system.

As a result of these and other changes, practitioners need education that prepares them to allocate limited resources skillfully, assume a wide range of diverse roles, and generate creative solutions in response to the demands of a dynamic, increasingly complex work environment.

Academic fieldwork coordinators are therefore faced with the challenge of making innovative changes to the traditional fieldwork model. The part-time therapist/full-time student (PTT/FTS) pilot study is an opportunity to engage students in a creative placement model that allows opportunities for self-directed learning and independence. In addition, the model uses occupational therapy practitioners in part-time positions who may otherwise not consider serving as educators for students in full-time placements. In the study, part-time practitioners assumed the fieldwork education and supervision of full-time students. Students were asked to document their experiences while taking part in placements where the fieldwork educator was a part-time occupational therapy practitioner available on a limited basis ranging from 10 to 30 hr/week. Researchers hoped that the students' written accounts of the challenges they encountered and the strategies they used to overcome them would provide insight into the specific types of learning experiences that are available to students during placements. Additionally, journal entries were expected to identify some of the essential features of the PTT/FTS model.

Method

Participants

Participants were 14 occupational therapy students from four universities placed at 12 sites for 4 to 8 weeks to complete their first, intermediate, or final field-work placement (see Table 1). Placement selection followed standard protocol; students chose situations that met their educational needs. Only researchers directly involved in evaluating journal material had access to the identities of participants. Selected journal entries were reproduced in reports with the journal authors' written consent and contained no identifying information. In addition, students were assured that participation (or nonparticipation) in the study would not affect the evaluation of their performance during placement.

Table 1
Student Participants in Part-Time Therapist/Full-Time Student Placements

University	Placement Sites	Placement		
		Length (weeks)	Number	Number of Students
McMaster University	Geriatric day hospital	6	4th	3
	Amputee program	5 to 6	Final	3
	Rheumatic disease unit	4	1st	1
University of Toronto	Work evaluation or hardening	8	Final	3
	Community geriatric program	5 and 8	3rd	4
	Geriatric program unit			
The University of Western Ontario	Mental health, child			
	Pediatrics (school system)			
	Pediatrics (children's center)			
University of Ottawa	Pediatrics (university research clinic)			
	Physical medicine and surgery			
	Geriatric evaluation unit			
	Upper-extremity and hand program			

Procedure

The criteria for selecting sites for PTT/FTS placements were limited to the following. A facility was required to have an occupational therapy practitioner who worked on site between 10 and 30 hr/week who was willing to accept a student for fieldwork education and to make arrangements for a second occupational therapy practitioner to be available to the student in case of emergencies when the primary practitioner was not working. Before placement, students received three blank journal notebooks with three postage-paid return envelopes and the following written instructions:

1. Keep a journal every other day on four questions: What were your main activities for the day, including contacts with your educator, other staff members, and clients? What did you learn, and what skills and knowledge were you able to demonstrate through these activities? Did you have any problems, and how were they resolved? What are your reflections on how the particular model used for your placement is working in practice?

2. Write a brief account of expectations before beginning the placement, an hour-by-hour log of daily activities every fourth entry, a detailed account of one case at mid-placement, and reflections on the overall placement experience in the last entry.

3. Use notebooks 1, 2, and 3 to record entries for weeks 1 and 2, weeks 3 and 4, and weeks 5 to 8 weeks, respectively, and return each notebook by mail at the end of each period.

The journal for 1 of the 14 students was not returned. Eleven participants sent back complete journals, and 2 participants returned journals with journal entries for only the first half of the placement. The journal for 1 of these participants mainly consisted of posthoc reports (i.e., the student indicated in the journal that all journal entries were written after the placement was completed) of tasks completed during the first half of the placement, and these data were excluded from the analysis. The data from the other participant's incomplete journal were used because the student appeared to be a "negative case" (Lincoln & Guba, 1985). However, because analysis can only be completed on journal entries for the first half of this practicum, researchers are uncertain if the students' attitudes changed in the second half of the placement, and thus the usefulness of this data is limited. One of the 11 complete sets of journals was written in French and translated to English for evaluation.

The journals were assembled at a central location, photocopied, and grouped by university for evaluation. The methodology guiding the journal analysis included two qualitative approaches: the constant comparative method of analysis (Glaser, 1978; Glaser & Strauss, 1967) and development of categories and themes (Lincoln & Guba, 1985). These strategies for evaluating qualitative data involve a circular process where broad concepts and categories are identified and then repeatedly recoded and recategorized with the aim of consolidating related elements of data into themes.

Journal evaluation was a three-step process. First, an academic occupational therapy fieldwork coordinator and a research assistant with a background in psychology independently reviewed photocopies of the student journals. Evaluators read the content of individual journal entries and coded text believed to be potentially part of an emerging theme. Elements of text with perceived similarities were hand sorted and grouped under the heading of an appropriate theme. Second, evaluators compared coded journal photocopies page-by-page to determine if any features of their interpretations matched. Comparison results generally fell into one of two categories.

1. Jointly identified themes with jointly identified groups of coded text

2. Different theme names with jointly coded groups of text

The procedure was applied to all journals with the journals of students from the same university evaluated in sequence. Third, the photocopies were clipped into individual units of coded text, which were then grouped according to how closely they fit with one of the emerging themes. Because some quotes contained elements of more than one theme, or were not clearly representative of an identified theme, the process served as a guide for reorganizing the data into more precisely defined categories. Data were resorted with the results of the previous sort as criteria until two categories of quotes emerged.

1. Those that fit reasonably well with an established theme or category

2. Those largely unrelated to themes, categories, or each other

Results and Discussion

Journal analysis identified distinct themes related to various aspects of the PTT/FTS model. In the following pages, these themes are illustrated by using direct quotes from student journals. Overall, when reviewing the student journals, it is apparent that one of the most important challenges that student participants faced was to generate learning opportunities during periods when the part-time educator was unavailable. This proved to be especially difficult when caseloads were limited.

In the student journals, three broad strategies to overcome the limitation of a lower caseload inherent in PTT/FTS placements are identified. For the purpose of this study, the strategies have been labeled *invited learning*, *delegated direct service*, and *strategy of multiple roles*.

Invited Learning

In invited learning, the students explored areas of interest within the placement setting and initiated learning relationships with health care professionals employed at the facility (Figure 1). In this strategy, the student initially invited himself or herself along to observe other practitioners at the site.

■ Informant 226: "[names practitioner] has it set up so that when she is here, we do everything together and when she isn't, I observe other programs at [names facility] with other OTs [occupational therapists] and other therapists (art, music). I like this because I can get a better idea of how the activities and programs are carried out for the children."

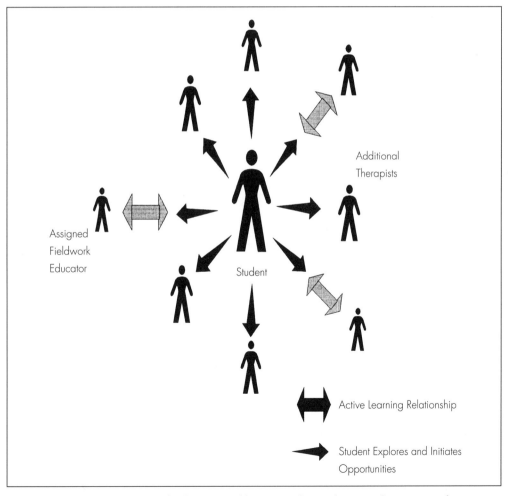

Figure 1. In the strategy identified as invited learning, the students explore areas of interest within the placement setting and initiate learning relationships with health care professionals employed at the facility.

■ Informant 401: "Contact with other OTs on my supervisor's day off has permitted me to gain a variety of OT experience in other sections and specialties."

Students often reported using invited learning strategies that incorporated hands-on practice and provided opportunities for active learning that continued throughout the entire placement. Invited learning was seen as an effective strategy by students, but some practitioners did not believe it was a legitimate way to handle the PTT/FTS model.

■ Informant 104: "I was fortunate enough to have two OTs take me under their wing so to speak...this stage in my learning, hands on with clients is the best way I can apply what I have learned in school....She [refers to the supervising practitioner] feels that what I have been doing is not a true reflection of part-time therapist supervision."

In addition to using the invited learning strategy with same discipline supervisors, students formed learning relationships with professionals from other disciplines. They described these types of learning situations as positive experiences.

■ Informant 105: "...the physio [therapist] on the team was great in terms of explaining what she was doing and answering all of my questions. It also gave me the opportunity to talk with them on an informal basis—this is a good opportunity."

■ Informant 214: "I've had to speak with other professionals other than OT for input since there were no other OTs here. This really helped me to recognize the vast knowledge base of other professions and how much an OT can gain by working collaboratively with them."

Delegated Direct Service

In this strategy, care of the fieldwork educator's clients is delegated to the student when the practitioner is off duty. Students often described handling the part-time practitioner's caseload on days when the practitioner worked, and then continuing to see patients on their own when the practitioner was not working.

■ Informant 401: "Having been advised by my OT supervisor, I had the opportunity to also conduct treatment of my OT's patients on her day off....The OT discussed my planned activities with patients for tomorrow. I plan to conduct an HDS cognitive assessment, fit a patient with clothes for a home visit, and observe a patient working on a computer."

Strategy of Multiple Roles

When the part-time practitioner was not present, students explored roles other than direct service. The alternative activities described by most students were related to research and education.

- Informant 103: "I had to reorganize my day. I reviewed the chart carefully and took some notes, I explored the library in the hospital, I had a chance to start my learning contract (that's early!), and I talked to my fellow student regarding the potential site visit we are going to pay."

- Informant 401: "I scheduled activities for tomorrow: I would like to complete my Orientation Checklist, review a patient's chart in detail, and do some research on Guillain-Barré syndrome."

The strategy of multiple roles was often identified within journal entries, but students did not seem to value it as much as direct client care.

- Informant 401: "...I have been very comfortable with deciding to visit patients instead of conducting research—something I could do on my own time, after office hours."

Emerging Themes

Journal analysis identified several themes that describe some essential features of the PTT/FTS model. These themes—time away, effective student–practitioner communication, self-direction, flexibility, and freedom to try the profession—will be described below with student quotes serving as illustration. The themes time away and effective student–practitioner communication describe features of the PTT/FTS model that can affect the student's placement experience in either a positive or negative way.

Time Away

The journal entries of students often describe the positive effect of spending large amounts of time away or apart from the practitioner. When the time available for student–fieldwork educator interaction is limited, the student and practitioner come to meetings prepared to get things done, and communication focuses on what is important. Time away provides students with an opportunity to practice independent problem solving and to rehearse newly acquired skills or reflect on learning between feedback meetings. The increase in student reflection that seems to accompany an increase in the level of independence that students are allowed during placements is a theme identified by Bossers, Cook, Polatajko, and Laine (1997) in a study of placements where student participants developed a role for occupational therapy in a community agency and received 3 to 5 hr of weekly education and supervision from an off-site occupational therapy practitioner.

In a similar manner, the following student quotes highlight the theme of time away for students engaging in the PTT/FTS placement.

- Informant 401: "A PTT/FTS placement also gives the student and the supervisor an appropriate 'time-out' from each other, and I believe that this breathing space allows the student and therapist to use their time together in a highly productive way, ensuring that personal contact does not become stale from over exposure. During my own time, I am able to recap my placement experiences, reflect on what has been learned, and reorganize and orient myself, by scheduling and planning, to move forward."

- Informant 213: "In some ways, this PTT/FTS model has been better. Not having 5-day per week contact with my supervisor provides me with more time to reflect on and evaluate my learning experience…having more time without direct supervision encouraged me to do more problem solving on my own, because my supervisor was not as readily available to answer questions."

Although students wrote of the positive effects of time away, they experienced some frustration.

- Informant 213: "The only drawbacks that I have experienced during this practicum are that most lunch breaks were scheduled for meetings with the supervising therapist because there was no other times available in her schedule. Also, I was sometimes frustrated by the delays in submitting reports because my supervising therapist needed to sign them but was not available to do so immediately. It is my opinion that these are small sacrifices, compared with the other gains I've made in this placement."

- Informant 104: "…talked with preceptor regarding the events of week. Clarified a few things. Finding it a bit frustrating that we're not having time for feedback. She leaves at 3:15 on the 3 days she is in."

Participants tended to report that the effect of time away was positive when the educator provided the student with structure and support without being too restrictive.

- Informant 401: "A key to the success of a PTT/FTS placement will not only be the willingness of the student to take on activities but also the actions and attitude of supervising therapists….By having sessions necessarily scheduled at fixed times according to the OT's working days, students are provided with concrete feedback, and this somewhat formal assessment allows students to modify behavior accordingly, on a regular basis."

Effective Student–Practitioner Communication

Not unlike other fieldwork situations (Christie, Joyce, & Moeller, 1985; Hummell, 1994; Mitchell & Kampfe, 1990), communication between the student and practitioner educator was identified as a key factor in determining the success of placements. Student journals identified the importance of good communication between the student and other practitioners who participated actively in the invited learning strategy.

- Informant 213: "The rapport that my supervising therapist and I had was critical to the success of this practicum. She felt comfortable with me working independently, knowing that I would call if necessary. I felt comfortable calling her. This mutual trust depended largely on my conscientious work habits. I always kept the supervising therapist informed of what I was doing or planned to do...the fact that I am able to determine what is pertinent information prevented me from making a lot of irrelevant calls to my supervising therapist on her days off."

- Informant 105: "...a big determinant of how well this model works out is definitely based on how well the two parties communicate with one another. Fortunately, my preceptor and I are open to meeting at least once a day."

Self-Direction

The importance of student self-direction was illustrated in the journal entries of a student who appeared to have been given a limited role in determining her learning needs. When a task with another discipline was assigned, the student believed that there would have been other better matched learning opportunities on site.

- Informant 338: "...though I did ask to have the opportunity to do some work in this area, I was suddenly TOLD that there were 8 voc. evals for me to do in April...this was communicated by [names another discipline] without even asking me how much I wanted to be involved!"

Flexibility

Student flexibility and self-direction both emerged as substrategies necessary for making invited learning and delegated direct service effective. Students described problem solving and exercising caution and judgment in decision making with client programs.

- Informant 401: "When given direction by OTs, I have felt competent to carry out their instructions and have been able to problem-solve easily when I've run into complications, in which circumstances, I have enjoyed the challenge....I feel an appropriate level of caution about performing activities that present a safety risk (example: transfers). In general, I have followed my schedule of planned activities, but I have been willing to make changes. For instance, I have replaced one activity with another when there was a cancellation, with no feelings of anxiety about doing this."

Freedom To Try the Profession

Within the PTT/FTS model, students described having the freedom to try the profession on days when the part-time practitioner was off-site.

- Informant 401: "On my days without supervision, I have a sense of what it might be like to be a qualified OT."

Although the experience of having the freedom to explore the profession and exposure to the reality of practice are to some extent inherent in all fieldwork placements, the students' subjective perceptions of their placement experiences, as described in their journals, indicated that they believe they gain a better understanding of entry-level practice in PTT/FTS placements than in traditional models due to having the opportunity to be more independent.

- Informant 214: "This placement has also been good for me as there isn't always an OT here to model. This has allowed me to feel more free in developing my own style."

Journal entries indicated that, as placements progressed, students became increasingly more independent. This independence was usually accompanied by an emerging sense of self-confidence.

- Informant 215: "I also learned that I can accomplish the goals I set out for myself...since I am in control of my own time, I feel confident I can meet these goals."

- Informant 105: "Furthermore, I completed a home assessment on Friday. I completed it independently and made a few recommendations in the end as I went along."

Students who became accustomed to being independent described having to readjust to working with the practitioner on the days that she was on-site.

- Informant 104: "It's always a bit of a readjustment on Tuesdays to get used to having her back and doing meetings with her—not independently."

Students expect more independence in the PTT/FTS. One participant wrote of the disappointment when the expected independence did not materialize.

- Informant 338: "...the placement...so far...has been quite disappointing...I can happily work on my own...but don't feel I have the freedom to do so yet."

Implications for Education

The strategies and themes identified in this pilot study delineate some of the positive characteristics of the PTT/FTS model. The strategies students used to cope with low caseloads and the limited availability of their preceptors may have inherent value for educating occupational therapy students.

Invited learning, delegated direct service, and the strategy of multiple roles may provide a way for individual students to fully use the educational opportunities of each placement setting. As student participants applied these strategies within the placement setting, they seemed to focus intuitively on areas of practice that were appropriate for their particular stage of development and to gain insight into their own learning needs as they acquired professional knowledge. In addition, the journal entries of students suggest that the process of identifying and acquiring essential practice knowledge within the fieldwork environment may help to enhance the development of students' professional identity. Time away appears to facilitate effective practitioner–student communication, allow students to consolidate learning, and promote the development of problem solving and reflection. The extensive freedom to try out the profession inherent in the PTT/FTS model may permit students to gain a more authentic understanding of the professional role of an occupational therapy practitioner than more traditional placements. This model may allow senior students the opportunity to experience more independence in fieldwork and may inherently facilitate interactions appropriate in final-stage fieldwork, including increased independence and consolidation of learning (Sullivan & Bossers, 1998). In the pilot study, only one junior student completing a first placement was involved. This student described the benefit of using other occupational therapy practitioners in the facility in the invited learning strategy.

The negative themes that emerged through journal analysis do not appear to be related to serious problems with the PTT/FTS model. The informant who described disillusionment with her placement did not believe she had the opportunity to explore the learning environment or initiate learning relationships. When assigned to another discipline that did not seem relevant to her learning needs, she expressed frustration with the experience. In addition, several students who believed they did not have enough opportunity to consult with their educators expressed frustration. Providing stakeholders with information about the organizational framework of the PTT/FTS model so that students can explore opportunities for invited learning, delegated service, or engagement in multiple roles with the practitioner before placement may eliminate problems of this nature. The practitioner can consult with colleagues to determine the potential availability of health care professionals willing to serve as learning resources for students.

Student participants in the PTT/FTS model seemed to thrive when three key factors were present in appropriate proportions.

1. Autonomy (students need be able to direct their own learning and to function independently within the parameters of their assigned roles, especially with clients)
2. Ample opportunity for hands-on practice
3. A positive student–educator relationship (students need varying levels of educational instruction, guidance, and support from the fieldwork educator)

Strengths and Limitations

The qualitative analysis described in this article was performed on journal data that was originally collected to augment the quantitative evaluation method of another researcher (Hart, 1997) who sought to compare outcomes of students and practitioners involved in different models of fieldwork education and supervision. These models included the student as supervisor (a model where a student engages in learning how to be a fieldwork educator while completing his or her placement) (Bossers, Hartley, & Gage, 1997; Hopkins-Rosseel, Cox, Blais, Bossers, Jung, & Paterson, 1997), an interdisciplinary model (a model where students of various disciplines complete fieldwork focusing on the enhancement of interdisciplinary professional relationships and education) (Bossers, Beaton, Gage, Cox, & Pepper, 1998), and the PTT/FTS model (as described in this article).

Students were asked to keep a journal on key questions (see Methods). Some of these questions produced accounts of activities completed on placement rather than the perceptions and beliefs that students held regarding the experience. One question, however, "What are your reflections on how the particular model used for your practicum is working in practice?" allowed the researchers to gain an understanding of the perceptions of students with respect to the PTT/FTS model. In addition, the question "Did you have any problems, and how were they resolved?" provided data that examine problems and possible strategies for resolution. Students did not keep journals in a regimented form, and the journals, despite their original purpose and structure, contained rich data for further analysis. The qualitative study described in this article was initiated by the authors to understand the experience of the PTT/FTS from the learner's perspective.

Conclusion

The PTT/FTS pilot study explored the potential for using this placement model as a method of teaching various competencies within the existing fieldwork placement framework. The themes that emerged from student journals paint a broad picture of the PTT/FTS placement. Participants appeared to use the higher levels of student independence inherent in the model to create more opportunities for self-directed learning, reflection, and problem solving. The students spent much of their time initiating learning relationships with persons other than their primary fieldwork educator as they explored areas of interest within the placement setting. Students believed that the experience of participating in fieldwork on a more global level allowed them to gain insight into the professional role of an occupational therapy practitioner.

The PTT/FTS approach appears to offer several advantages. The highly flexible structure of the model can be adapted to a wide range of placement settings and shaped to fit the unique circumstances of persons who are participating in fieldwork education. In addition, the model's organizational framework provides a basis for developing a placement learning environment that inherently challenges students to take responsibility for fulfilling their own learning needs. The model likewise offers a way for students to use more fully the educational opportunities within each placement setting. However, the strengths of the model may be viewed negatively by students and practitioners who expect to work in a traditional full-time practitioner model. Educators must be aware that fieldwork sites, students, and practitioners may require support and information to properly implement this model. A handbook to support fieldwork educators, students, and other stakeholders has been developed to facilitate sites that want to implement the PTT/FTS model (Desrosiers, Bossers, Hartley, & Gage, 1997).

Further research will be required to evaluate more fully the role of part-time educators and the applicability of the PTT/FTS model in fieldwork education. A longer-term follow-up study examining the entry-level job performance of students who participate in placements with greater levels of independence would help to establish the effectiveness of this model. As health care evolves and new professional competencies begin to emerge, creative models of fieldwork education must be developed and implemented under the direction of experienced clinicians.

Acknowledgments

We thank the occupational therapy students, their fieldwork educators and supervisors, and the university faculty members who participated in the pilot projects. Their insights and innovative efforts have laid a solid foundation on which to build future placements with part-time fieldwork educators. We likewise recognize the contribution to this study of the following university faculty members who were involved with the PTT/FTS pilot projects: Arlene Anthony, Marcel Desrosiers, Barb Gaiptman, Marie Gage, Bonny Jung, Helene Polatajko, and Barbara Cooper.

References

Bossers, A. M., Beaton, C., Gage, M., Cox, P., & Pepper, J. (1998). Interdisciplinary clinical education in a rehabilitation setting: A pilot project. In *Abstracts of the 12th International Congress of the World Federation of Occupational Therapists* (Abstract No. 1422, B3–B13). Montreal, Quebec, Canada: WFOT.

Bossers, A. M., Cook, J. V., Polatajko, H. J., & Laine, C. (1997). Understanding the role-emerging fieldwork placement. *Canadian Journal of Occupational Therapy, 64*, 70–81.

Bossers, A. M., Desrosiers, M., Jung, B., Anthony, A., & Gage, M. (June, 1997). *The part-time therapist/full-time student fieldwork placement.* Paper was presented the Canadian Association of Occupational Therapists conference, Halifax, Nova Scotia, Canada.

Bossers, A. M., Hartley, M., & Gage, M. (1997). *Student as supervisor resource manual*. London, Ontario, Canada: The University of Western Ontario School of Occupational Therapy.

Christie, B., Joyce, P. C., & Moeller, P. C. (1985). Fieldwork experience. Part 2: The supervisor's dilemma. *American Journal of Occupational Therapy, 39*, 675–681.

Desrosiers, M., Bossers, A. M., Hartley, M., & Gage, M. (1997). *Part-time therapist/full-time student resource manual*. London, Ontario, Canada: University of Western Ontario School of Occupational Therapy.

Glaser, B. (1978). *Theoretical sensitivity: Advances in the methodology of grounded theory.* Mill Valley, CA: Sociology Press.

Glaser, B., & Strauss, A. (1967). *The discovery of grounded theory: Strategies for qualitative research*. New York: Aldine.

Hart, D. (1997). *Models of supervision: A discussion paper on the student exit survey results*. Unpublished manuscript, Ontario Institute of Education, University of Toronto, Ontario, Canada.

Hopkins-Rosseel, D., Cox, P., Blais, S., Bossers, A. M., Jung, B., & Paterson, M. (1997). The student as supervisor model of clinical education. *Canadian Physical Therapy Association National Congress, Physiotherapy Canada, 49*(2, Suppl. 5).

Hummell, J. (1994). Effective fieldwork supervision: The occupational therapy students' perspective. *Proceedings of the 11th International Congress of the World Federation of Occupational Therapists*, 408–410.

Lincoln, Y. S., & Guba, E. G. (1985). *Naturalistic inquiry*. Newbury Park, CA: Sage.

Mitchell, M. M., & Kampfe, C. M. (1990). Coping strategies used by occupational therapy students during fieldwork: An exploratory study. *American Journal of Occupational Therapy, 44*, 543–550.

Stanton, S. (1997). Catch the excitement. *National, 14*(1), 3.

Sullivan, T. M., & Bossers, A. M. (1998). Occupational therapy fieldwork levels. *National, 15*(3), 7–9.

Self-Directed Learning: A Model for Occupational Therapy Fieldwork

E. Adel Herge

Suzanne A. Milbourne

E. Adel Herge, MS, OTR/L, is Instructor, and Suzanne A. Milbourne, MS, OTR/L, is Adjunct Faculty Member, Thomas Jefferson University, Philadelphia, Pennsylvania.

Self-directed learning is one model of fieldwork supervision. This model trains future practitioners to be effective in alternative settings by using methods during fieldwork such as consultation, needs evaluation, program development, and evaluation. The model supports recognition of adult learner's life experiences and the adult learner's readiness to learn, and it facilitates development of professional and clinical skills. Additionally, the responsibility for learning is placed on the learner, and, in doing so, it encourages transition from classroom to clinics, which prepares fieldwork students for lifelong learning. Methods discussed include on-site supervision, off-site preceptor meetings, use of student and preceptor logs, and a trilinear learning contract.

T his article will describe the self-directed learning (SDL) model and its application to the adult learner and propose the usefulness of the model in occupational therapy fieldwork education. Application of the model to Level I fieldwork experiences for students in community-based, nontraditional settings will be discussed.

Purpose of Fieldwork Education

Fieldwork education provides the opportunity for the occupational therapy student to integrate academic theory with clinical practice. Through the fieldwork experience, the occupational therapy student develops knowledge, values, and therapeutic skills under the careful eye of the supervising practitioner. In an effort to prepare today's students to be tomorrow's occupational therapy practitioners, fieldwork education has shifted from more traditional settings to community-based and nontraditional sites (Crist, 1997; Joe, 1998). Even in the more typical and traditional fieldwork sites, there has been a shift in training. Supervising practitioners often have less time to devote to student training (Crist, 1998), and students may be working in departments where direct supervision may not come from an occupational therapy practitioner.

The typical models of supervision, long practiced by experienced clinical supervisors, have had to give way to new and more innovative models to accommodate this change in clinical practice and fieldwork placement. This article will describe a model of clinical supervision formulated on the basis of SDL and will describe the authors' use of this model in Level I community-based fieldwork.

Traditional Models

Traditional models of fieldwork supervision have been built on the apprenticeship model or "learning by doing." In this model, students work closely with the supervising practitioner and gradually assume responsibility for clients on the practitioner's caseload. The student is expected to acquire the knowledge, skills, and values of the supervising practitioner by observing and modeling behavior. A limitation of this model is that students may not necessarily develop skills in independent critical analysis, clinical reasoning, and creative problem solving.

SDL

Knowles (1975) developed the concept of SDL. He defined it as a dynamic process in which the learner reaches out to incorporate new experiences, relates present situations with previous experiences, and reorganizes current experiences on the basis of this process. In this model, the learner is responsible for identifying his or her learning needs and for developing a strategy to meet those needs. The learner, rather than the teacher, is responsible for the learning process. This differs from the more traditional teacher-directed model in which the teacher is responsible for setting educational goals, selecting content and determining how it will be presented, and evaluating whether goals have been met. Knowles (1975) stated that the SDL model is more useful in adult learning, which he refers to as *andragogy*. This approach differs from the learning of children, *pedagogy*, in several ways. In pedagogical learning, the instructor makes decisions regarding content and pacing of learning material. In contrast, the andragogical approach recognizes that the student is coming to the learning situation with history and experience. The adult learner is perceived to be autonomous and self-directed, thereby reducing the conflict that often arises when the adult learner is placed in a position of dependence on the "teacher." The pedagogical model assumes the learner is ready to learn on the basis of age or the completion of prerequisite material, which simulates a developmental model. In the andragogical model, readiness to learn is attributed to the need or desire to develop greater skill or competence. Material is organized and present-ed in a logical order in the pedagogical model of learning. An andragogical model focuses on a problem-centered approach, believing that the learning will be more meaningful if related to relevant experiences. External rewards such as grades or competition motivate the pedagogical learner. By contrast, the adult learner responds to a sense of internal reward such as the feeling of accomplish-ment one has from mastering a new technique or skill.

The SDL model has been used in business, industry, nursing, medical, and pharmacy education (Hardigan, 1994; Knowles et al., 1984; Martens, 1981; Wiley, 1983). Proponents of this model suggest that professional education must include not only the transmission of knowledge, attitudes, and skills but also should focus on the skills of inquiry and the process of learning. Theoretically, habits of lifelong learning develop with this model. One example is that of med-ical school education. Knowles et al. (1984) believed that professional education of physicians should produce "physicians who are able to assess changing health care needs, keep up with changing concepts and new knowledge, and adapt their own performance accordingly" (p. 210).

SDL Models in Occupational Therapy

A literature review describes the limited use of SDL in occupational therapy fieldwork education. Gaiptman and Anthony (1989) described the use of this model as a framework for clinical education. Mickan (1995) used the model in the development of a learning packet for use with students preparing for a specialty fieldwork placement in pediatrics. It is of interest to the authors that both of these articles are from outside the United States.

SDL in Level I Fieldwork Education

A major task for university, college, and clinical educators is to prepare students to meet the demands of 21st-century practice. Such challenges include negotiating the changing health care system, working in nontraditional community-based settings, developing collaborative relationships with colleagues outside the traditional sphere (Baum, 1997), and entering practice confident in one's abilities to meet new and unforeseen challenges. A recent American Occupational Therapy Association study indicated that 24% of newly registered occupational therapy practitioners are working in community-based settings (Steib, 1996). In many of the settings, practitioners work independently, with minimal supervision, or with cross-discipline supervision.

In 1994, the Occupational Therapy Department at Thomas Jefferson University (Philadelphia, PA) began placing students in Level I fieldwork settings with off-site occupational therapy preceptors providing supervision. It became clear that traditional, apprenticeship models of supervision were inadequate for students in these settings because no occupational therapy practitioners were on-site. Therefore, we began to search for a framework for developing a supervision model on the basis of a set of beliefs (see Table 1).

Application of Model

As stated earlier, in the SDL model, the learner is responsible to identify their learning needs and to develop a strategy for meeting those needs. It is important to note that, when we applied this model to fieldwork experiences, the underlying structure of the experience was built on the course syllabus objectives. University guidelines and procedures for course work were maintained, and the students completed the same assignments as non-SDL supervised peers. Students were required to complete course assignments and meet course content requisites. The SDL model provided a framework for promoting independence in settings that were nontraditional.

Table 1
Supervision Framework

Belief	Support	Projected Outcome
Fieldwork is an opportunity to develop professional as well as technical skills.	Foto (1997) stated that successful occupational therapy practitioners of the future will function in non-traditional environments, work in "self-managed" teams, and be critical thinkers.	We wanted to use the fieldwork experience as an opportunity to develop these skills. The SDL model is one strategy supporting this outcome.
Adult learners should be recognized for their life experiences and readiness to learn.	Knowles (1975) stated that the rich life experiences adult learners bring to the learning stituation enhances their readiness to learn.	We believed that fieldwork experiences in a somewhat unstructured setting would stimulate the student's readiness and motivation to apply concepts introduced through university coursework—a sort of "do or die" approach.
Emphasis for learning should be placed on the learner.	Christ (1997) reported that students who successfully complete fieldwork are those who are assertive, active learners who are interested, motivated, and engaged in the learning process.	Students must be autonomous and reflective in their thinking process and be able to "think on their feet" and respond immediately to a situation without the guidance of the supervising practitioner. Later, students must be able to reflect on the experience and follow-up with discussion with the preceptor.
Students need to transition from the classroom to clinics of the future.	Mickan (1995) viewed fieldwork as the opportunity to apply relevant knowledge to clinical practice.	We wanted to encourage our students to move from the teacher-directed classroom to the self-directed clinical setting.
Students need to prepare for lifelong learning.	Knowles (1984) believed that, to stay viable in health care of the future, students must develop habits of lifelong learning during professional education and training.	Students will identify their own learning needs and styles, select appropriate resources, and reflect on their personal and professional growth and development through the learning process.

Fieldwork settings selected included an outpatient methadone program for pregnant women in substance abuse recovery, an inpatient substance abuse recovery program for mothers and their children, and a community-based day program for adults with developmental disabilities. The settings were located in a large inner city, a low socioeconomic status suburban community, and a suburban industrial center, respectively. All three centers were eager and willing to offer student training and designated an on-site, facility staff supervisor.

Student selection for the fieldwork settings took into account both objective and subjective information gathered during the student's first year of enrollment in the occupational therapy program. Martens (1981) suggested that SDL is most appropriate for students nearing completion of their academic coursework. Only second-year students were eligible; however, we selected from both bachelor's degree- and master's degree-level students. Through a student interest survey administered by the fieldwork coordinator, students provided information about their research and clinical interests. Preference was given to students with interests in pediatrics, mental health, or community-based practice. Subjective information included faculty member verbal reports of student in-class interpersonal skills and judgments made regarding the maturity level of the student.

The model consists of five tools or techniques to support student supervision. Each are described in terms of the rationale for use and the method in which we used it.

On-Site Supervision

All three on-site, non-occupational therapy supervisors were professionals designated by the facility to supervise the students. They were specialists in a particular domain of clinical practice, either substance abuse, child development, or adults with developmental delays. Two of the settings have a history of supervising multidiscipline fieldwork students; this was the first experience for the third setting. The on-site supervisor served as a role model and resource for the students while on-site. He or she helped students focus on programmatic issues such as scheduling, assignments, expectations, and professional boundaries. The on-site supervisor provided clinical expertise regarding the specific population with whom they worked.

Off-Site Preceptor Meetings

Two faculty members from the university precepted the selected students. Mandatory group preceptor meetings were held on campus two to three times per month, usually for 1 to 2 hr. Both students and preceptors logged these meetings, and the time spent at each meeting counted toward required fieldwork time. Time spent in the preceptor meetings was emphasized as being as equally important as the time spent on site. According to Knowles et al. (1984), such meetings represent a laboratory of learning about human interactions where students can develop interpersonal skills and become aware of their own emotional reactions to new and unfamiliar situations. The meetings focused on student presentation of issues faced at the fieldwork site, their questions and concerns, and group problem solving.

Student Clinical Logs

This is a familiar technique often used in fieldwork experiences. This process of recording has been shown in the literature to enhance self-reflection and provides evidence of clinical reasoning growth and development (Sedlak, 1992). We selected this tool for three reasons.

1. It encourages self-reflection.
2. It serves as a basis for dialogue with the preceptor.
3. It encourages active learning.

The required 1/2-page log was expanded for the selected students to record a deeper reflection of their daily experiences at the clinical site. The log then served as a mechanism for dialogue. Each week, students turned in a copy of their log to their off-site preceptor, and the log served as a basis for discussion at the preceptor meetings. Active learning was encouraged in that students lead group discussions that focused on their learning needs or objectives. Additionally, the logs helped the students to become aware their learning styles.

Preceptor Logs

Off-site preceptors likewise kept a log of experiences during this supervision process. These served as a basis for our own self-reflection because this process was new to us as well as the students. Preceptors who reflect on their own learning experience possess a rich resource for discovering ways to be more helpful to the learner's reflection process. Additionally, logs enhance collaboration skills by using reflective information for dialog and discussion and, in turn, facilitate one's learning (Cooper, 1980). Finally, the preceptor clinical log provides concrete longitudinal data to support, modify, and objectify the development of this supervision process.

Trilinear Learning Contracts (TLC)

In the literature, the learning contract is described as a written agreement between teacher and student that itemizes what the learner will do to achieve specified learning outcomes. Creation of a learning contract is a process in which the "individual takes initiative in diagnosing their learning needs, formulating learning goals, identifying human and material resources for learning, choosing and implementing appropriate learning strategies, and evaluating learning outcomes" (Knowles, 1975, p. 18). Researchers have identified characteristics of students who complete this process, including self-reflection, creativity, motivation for learning, self-discipline, autonomy in learning, development of habits related to lifelong learning and professional development, and a sense of competence (Jennett, 1992).

Traditionally, the learning contract includes 4 parts; however, after 2 semesters, the university faculty members adapted the traditional learning contract and created the TLC. The authors selected the title *TLC* because the contract became a written agreement between the preceptor (faculty member), the student, and the on-site supervisor. Therefore, the TLC was modified to include 6 parts (Table 2).

Usefulness of the SDL Model

To determine the usefulness of using the SDL model, the authors reviewed the comments of the on-site supervisors, the preceptor clinical logs, and students' feedback. The authors acknowledge this data as preliminary.

On-Site Supervisor

Informal meetings and telephone conversations resulted in positive responses from the on-site supervisors. They indicated that, compared with other students at the setting, the students being supervised with the SDL model came to the

Table 2
Trilinear Learning Contract

Components	Description
Objectives	The student spends time diagnosing their own learning needs and translating them into objectives.
Learning resources and strategies	The student suggests resources to support completion of objectives and a means of accessing the resources.
Evidence of accomplishment	The student identifies behaviors that demonstrate completed learning objectives and what behaviors to evaluate.
Timeline	Due to the short time spent in the fieldwork setting, students needed to be encouraged to forge ahead more quickly in creating their objectives and spend a greater amount of time carrying these out in a timely manner.
Off-site preceptor role	The preceptor's roles are clarified as well as the expectation for and of the student.
On-site supervisor role	Including the on-site supervisor in this contracting and learning process, the authors hoped to increase their interest and commitment to this process rather than viewing their role as merely providing a fieldwork placement.

fieldwork site with a focus, were flexible and adaptable, and were able to work independently.

Preceptor Clinical Logs

Self-directed models of teaching enhance a student's critical thinking skills, ability to define goals, and manage time effectively. Students become flexible in practice and exhibit a personal, lifelong commitment to learning (Jennett, 1992). On the basis of the authors' observations, learning increased as the supervision process unfolded over the course of a semester. Students moved from passive participation to initiation and became leaders of group meetings. For a few students, self-confidence evolved and improved, which was exhibited by their ability to initiate communication and collaboration with on-site staff members. Anxiety about "What is my role? What is the role of occupational therapy in this setting?" decreased as seen in the students' ability to articulate gaps or opportunities for occupational therapy intervention at their fieldwork setting. Interpersonal skills and the ability to be culturally sensitive improved, as demonstrated in the students' clinical logs and group discussions. Improvement in the ability to problem solve and access resources for support or clarification of situations was demonstrated in the students' presentation of possible solutions rather than asking for answers. Finally, conceptual thinking skills emerged and were refined, for example, when the students articulated the uniqueness of occupational therapy and the contributions the profession may bring to a particular facility.

Student's Reactions to the SDL Model

Jennifer. "When my partner and I first received our blank learning contract, I remember feeling somewhat lost. We were going to a nontraditional setting, working with an unfamiliar population in the community, with no OT present to hold our hand along the way. To say the least, the ambiguity was somewhat unsettling. As a Level I student, all I longed for was structure. I felt like—tell me what to do, when to do it, how to document it, and lastly tell me what I will learn from the experience.

"Despite my initial apprehension, I began to work on my contract and really begin to think about what I wanted to learn and develop and how I was going to reach those objectives. It began to focus my thinking into what I needed to gain first, before I could move on the next step....I wanted to be able to keep a somewhat cohesive focus for treatment, without duplicating the other disciplines....In short, the learning contract allowed me to really think about what I wanted to gain/develop and how I was going to provide evidence to myself and to my preceptor that I was learning what I intended to. It also allowed me to think about what would be realistic and achievable with in the limited time frame of my clerkship.

"This self-directed learning process allowed my partner and me to develop our own individual objectives, even though we were working toward the same ultimate goal. In my opinion, this added to our creativity and the effectiveness of our end product because we were coming from a slightly different angle and knowledge base. Using the learning contract helped to facilitate autonomy….It helped me to develop confidence in my decisions because I had to decide for myself what I was trying to gain and how I was going to prove it. Although I'm not currently using a learning contract in my Level II experience, I use the thinking process a lot to guide my own self-directed learning. There are many times when I have to figure out how I'm going to meet my own objectives clinically, as well as how my patients are going to meet their objectives. More importantly, how will I know that my goals are met and that my efforts are directed in the right place? Using it as a guide allows me to take into account my own learning style, while also allowing me to take into account the differences among my patients.

"A couple of weeks ago, I asked one of my patients who is diagnosed with depression one simple question. I said, 'How will you know when you feel better?' She replied, 'What do you mean? I'll just know because I'll just feel better.' I then had her write down everything that would show or prove that she was feeling better. She compiled a list of things like "1. I will have more energy to put on make-up and do my hair. 2. I will get out of the house to run errands," etc. It was helpful to have something tangible for both of us to be able to document progress. It also was empowering for her to feel in control of the objective of her treatment.

"In looking back on my experience at [the fieldwork site] and the process of the self-directed learning, that is the first time I remember feeling like I was finally beginning to think like an OT. Ironically enough, it was in a nontraditional setting where there was doubt that an OT even belonged."

Carla. "During my last Level I affiliation, I was introduced to the 'learning contract.' This contract required me to determine what I wanted to learn from my clerkship, how I was going to go about finding the information, and how I was going to determine if I had learned what I wanted to learn. At first I said to myself "Great, more work for me to do." After I completed the contract, I realized that it was going to be beneficial to my learning experience. It made me think about what I wanted to achieve while working at the site. It also gave me measurable goals to strive for. I wasn't a passive player in my educational experience. I was able to play an active role."

Suggestions for future application of this model include

■ comparison studies examining effectiveness of this model versus other supervision models in community-based settings,

■ comparison of student performance in similar settings with different supervision models,

■ expansion of this model for use in other professional training programs, and

■ training of clinical educators in use of the SDL model.

Conclusion

Current challenges in occupational therapy clinical practice and fieldwork education require the development of new models of supervision. Issues facing clinical educators include decreased supervision time, use of non-occupational therapy supervisors, lack of sufficient sites, increase in community-based sites, and changing practice. Issues facing academic educators include preparing students to enter clinical practice as reflective, autonomous, critical thinkers who are flexible and adaptive in practice and are creative problem solvers. The model described in this article provides one strategy to meet the needs of both clinical and academic educators as well as the demands of clinical practice. ■

Acknowledgments

This material has been previously presented in the following formats.

■ Herge, E. A., & Milbourne, S. A. (April, 1998). *Tri-linear learning contract and off-site fieldwork education.* Poster session presented at the annual conference of the American Occupational Therapy Association, Baltimore, MD.

■ Milbourne, S. A., & Herge, E. A. (1998, May 21). Fieldwork supervision using TLC. *OT Week,12*(21), www.*OTWeek*.org.

■ Milbourne, S. A., & Herge, E. A. (October, 1997). *An innovative approach to fieldwork supervision.* Paper presented at the state conference of the Pennsylvania Occupational Therapy Association, Mars, PA.

References

Baum, C. (1997). The managed care system: The educator's opportunity. *Education Special Interest Section Quarterly, 7*, 1–3.

Cooper, S. (1980). Problem-based learning and approach toward reforming allied health education. *Journal of Allied Health, 21*(3), 161–173.

Crist, P. (1997, June 16). How students "hit fieldwork running." *Advance, 13*(24), 4.

Crist, P. (1998, January 19). Fieldwork in the new millennium. *Advance, 14*(3), 5, 29.

Foto, M. (1997). Preparing occupational therapists for the year 2000: The impact of managed care on education and training. *American Journal of Occupational Therapy, 51*, 88–90.

Gaiptman, B., & Anthony, A. (1989). Contracting in fieldwork education: The model of self-directed learning. *Canadian Journal of Occupational Therapy, 56*(1), 10–14.

Hardigan, P. (1994). Investigation of learning contracts in pharmaceutical education. *American Journal of Pharmaceutical Education, 58*(4), 386–390.

Jennett, P. A. (1992). Self-directed learning: A pragmatic view. *Journal of Continuing Education in the Health Professions, 12*, 99–104.

Joe, B. E. (1998, February 19). Where have the clinicians gone? *OT Week, 12*(8), 14–15.

Knowles, M. (1975). *Self-directed learning: A guide for learners and teachers.* Chicago: Follett.

Knowles, M. & Associates (1984). *Andragogy in action.* San Francisco: Jossey-Bass.

Martens, K. (1981). Self-directed learning: An option for nursing education. *Nursing Outlook, 29*, 472–477.

Mickan, S. M. (1995). Student preparation for pediatric fieldwork. *British Journal of Occupational Therapy, 58*(6), 239–244.

Sedlak, C. (1992). Use of clinical logs by beginning nursing students and faculty to identify learning needs. *Journal of Nursing Education, 31*(1), 24–28.

Steib, P. A. (1996, May 23). The new OTRs: Who are they? *OT Week, 10*(20), 16–18.

Wiley, K. (1983). Effects of a self-directed learning project and preferences for structure on self-directed learning readiness. *Nursing Research, 32*(3), 181–185.

Student to Practitioner: The Adaptive Transition

Janette K. Schkade

Janette K. Schkade, PhD, OTR, FAOTA, is Professor and Dean, Texas Woman's University, School of Occupational Therapy, Denton, Texas.

This model was presented at the American Occupational Therapy Association Practice Conference in St. Louis, MO, 1996. It has been presented to fieldwork supervisors at University of North Dakota, Grand Forks, ND; Arapahoe Community College, Englewood, CO; Dominican College, Orangeburg, NY; Duquesne University, Pittsburgh, PA; and Texas Woman's University, Dallas, TX, and Houston, TX.

Fieldwork education is an essential part of the education of the occupational therapy practitioner. As the student makes the transition from classroom to clinic, both student and supervisor are faced with challenges that are exacerbated by today's health care environments. This article presents a model of student transition on the basis of the occupational adaptation frame of reference. By viewing the transition from classroom to clinic as one example of normal professional development, this model provides a structure that can be used by both student and supervisor to understand and facilitate the developmental process.

T he transition from classroom to clinic or other intervention settings is one of a series of professional transitions in the occupational role of practitioner (Cohn, 1993; Cohn & Crist, 1995; Kramer & Stern, 1995; Schkade, 1991; Wiemer, 1991). In the author's experience as both a fieldwork educator and an academic educator, many students go through fieldwork with few problems. Some have only moderate and transitory difficulty. Yet others have extreme difficulty, which occasionally results in termination before fieldwork completion or a failing grade when the fieldwork is completed. To achieve the desired outcome of emerging competence in occupational functioning as a practitioner, the student must adapt to professional challenges that the workplace presents. Acquisition of this outcome requires mutual understanding and meaningful exchange of information and ideas on the part of both fieldwork educator and student. The model presented in this article is offered as one approach to understanding and facilitating the student development process. Its purpose is to provide a way to "name and frame" (Schon, 1983) behaviors students exhibit during this time of professional transition. In so doing, this model can give both the fieldwork educator and student a language with which to identify problem areas and discuss possible solutions. It can be useful for both occupational therapy and occupational therapy assistant students and educators.

The model is formulated on the basis of the occupational adaptation (OA) frame of reference (Schkade & Schultz, 1992; Schultz & Schkade, 1992). Briefly, OA assumes that competence in occupational functioning develops as the result of experiences in which the person engages an internal adaptation process. For reasons of parsimony, the person is seen as consisting of sensorimotor, cognitive, and psychosocial systems that are uniquely present in each person as a result of genetic or familial, environmental, and experiential or phenomenological influences. The OA process unfolds as follows.

1. The person, acting within an occupational role, responds to challenges by first perceiving the role expectations. Role expectations are a combination of internal and external expectations. In the case of the fieldwork student,

the challenges involve client evaluation and intervention as well as staff member and team interaction. The internal role expectations the students bring stem from their personal competence and their therapeutic competence. External expectations are those the facility contributes in the form of client population needs and facility needs.

2. To meet role expectations, the person generates a response, evaluates it, and integrates the outcome information for future use. This process allows the person to attempt adaptive responses and affect occupational functioning as a result. The fieldwork student develops an action, carries it out, evaluates its effectiveness, and makes adaptations as needed for improved functioning. The information in a particular event, whether positive or negative, is stored in the student's adaptive behavior repertoire for future use.

3. Those acting as agents of the occupational environment (i.e., the context in which the challenge occurs, uniquely configured by physical, social, and cultural influences) evaluate the outcomes and feed that information back into the environmental systems. Just as with the person, the information from a particular event has the potential to affect the environment and its expectations. As applied to the fieldwork case, the supervisors and members of the intervention team evaluate whether the student response met the facility expectations. This evaluation can lead those responsible for the student's education to modify role expectations in some way, either by easing some of the expectations or by intensifying them to promote student development while still meeting facility needs.

The OA construct on which the student model rests is the adaptive response behavior, a component of the adaptive response generation function. Adaptive response behaviors are classified as primitive, transitional, and mature. (The classification labels were influenced by Gilfoyle, Grady, & Moore [1990].) As used in OA, the classifications of primitive, transitional, and mature behaviors represent classes of behavior rather than a developmental progression. The behaviors are seen in sensorimotor, cognitive, and psychosocial systems. Table 1 presents a description of typical behaviors, causation, and action outcome for each class. The stimuli for these behaviors are embedded in the challenges with which the student is confronted, especially those that require new or newly differentiated response patterns.

Primitive behaviors are those that involve attempts by the student to stabilize an ego threatened by the possibility of a failure experience. Thus, the causal influence is perceived need for ego defense. The defenses used are the more primitive ones: denial, projection, and avoidance. These responses result in hyperstabilization of one or more of the person systems and thus represent a response that immobilizes rather than promotes mastery outcomes. The use of primitive behaviors as an initial reaction to an ego-threatening challenge is con-

Table 1
Adaptive Response Behaviors: Student Transition Model

Primitive	Transitional	Mature
Behaviors	*Behaviors*	*Behaviors*
Deny	Act without adequate	Initiate information seeking
Project	rationale (incomplete,	Problem solve
Avoid	illogical, or inaccurate)	Break set
		Think creatively
Causation	*Causation*	*Causation*
Defense of self	Activity as goal	Theory, goal, activity integration
Action outcome	*Action outcome*	*Action outcome*
Hyperstability	Hypermobility	Blended mobility
(immobilization)	(mobility without	and stability
	modulation)	(therapeutic and goal directed)

sidered normative. Such use allows the student an opportunity to regain equilibrium from which to begin adaptive movement. Thus, as a first response, primitive behavior can be part of a response pattern that is ultimately adaptive. If this type of behavior persists beyond the time needed for equilibrium restoration, the result will be interference with professional development and is considered dysadaptive.

Transitional behaviors reflect excessive movement or hypermobility in one or more person systems. When using transitional behaviors, the student acts without adequate rationale (i.e., behaviors result from cognitions or perceptions that are largely incomplete, illogical, or inaccurate). The causal influence is the perception of activity as goal. Hypermobile responses reflect action for the sake of being active. These responses lack modulation present in true goal-directed response. The student with transition behaviors may act with a "do something even if it's wrong" attitude because there is an understanding that some action is required. Transitional behaviors are more promising. Unlike the primitive behaviors, transitional behaviors demonstrate variability. The activity can allow the supervisor to see behaviors that are appropriate to reinforce or facilitate. Thus, attempts at mastery present in transitional behaviors are characterized by mobility without the modulation necessary for true goal direction.

Mature student behaviors are those said to be driven by blending stability and mobility attributes. As with primitive and transitional behaviors, mature behaviors can be seen in all person systems. These behaviors incorporate information seeking, problem solving, creative thinking, and the ability to break perceptual set. When problem-solving approaches are used, the student takes responsibility for initiating skill development efforts. Thus, the adaptation process is functioning at an optimal level. The potential for mastery, generalization to other tasks, and self-initiation of new adaptations in response to subsequent challenges is at its strongest.

It should be noted that the student might operate at all behavior levels from primitive to mature. All three classes of behavior remain in the student's repertoire. Furthermore, there is no immutable sequence in which the behaviors occur. The more competent student will spend less time in primitive and transitional behaviors, whereas the less competent student will typically spend more time demonstrating these behaviors and may exhibit few or none of the mature behaviors. When confronted with a new challenge that seems overwhelming at the outset, even the relatively competent student may resort to more primitive behaviors as a temporary balance-restoring strategy. The optimal outcome is that successively less time and effort are expended in primitive behaviors and that, with subsequent challenges, more rapid movement to mature behaviors develops.

It is important to emphasize that sensorimotor, cognitive, and psychosocial systems are present in every response. The holistic nature of the theory on which this model is based requires such a perspective. To separate responses by system is inherently artificial because the behavior invariably integrates the system, whether the response is functional or dysfunctional. However, it is useful to momentarily isolate the behaviors by system as a way to better identify and think about them. When problem behaviors arise, identification of a focal point can lead to discussion between fieldwork educator and student about how to facilitate adaptive change. This can be particularly useful when a problem seems diffuse and difficult to remediate.

Sensorimotor System

The sensorimotor system involves abilities to respond to tasks that require perceptual-motor responses such as those required in administering evaluations, physically handling patients or clients, fabricating orthoses or assistive devices, manipulating materials and equipment, and so forth.

Primitive behaviors, which reflect hyperstability, may be physically removing oneself from the task, complaining of illness, or other attempts to avoid sensorimotor demands. Handling of the patient may be so intensive that it immobilizes the patient rather than facilitates movement. Rigid or defensive postures can connote primitive sensorimotor behaviors.

Transitional sensorimotor behaviors manifest as active but are not truly goal-directed. Handling the patient may involve eliciting movement for the sake of eliciting movement without awareness of dysfunctional patterns. Handling may appear overly aggressive. Measurement devices or orthoses may be reversed, inverted, or otherwise placed in a manner suggesting random sensorimotor activity.

Mature behaviors are indicated by efforts to develop or practice requisite skills for a particular task. Awareness of how a patient is responding to handling and an adjustment to facilitate improved response if necessary are other indications. A type of coordinated and purposive fluidity in sensorimotor behavior can be seen.

Cognitive System

Challenges requiring cognitive system responses are those that tap knowledge bases regarding diagnosis, evaluation, or treatment. Reporting evaluation and intervention information in both oral and written forms is included.

Primitive cognitive responses once again reflect ego-defensive strategies. They reflect hyperstabilization or immobilization, which interfere with cognitive movement. Denial of prior exposure to certain conditions or complaints of incomplete exposure often occur. A "glazing over" of the eyes can be a manifestation. If the student is expected to participate in team rounds in the discussion of a patient or client, the primitive responses can be total silence, sometimes accompanied by a failure to make eye contact with any potential questioner. Retreat into excessive note taking is a common example of a cognitive system behavior that may have served the student well in another environment (academic and didactic courses). The perceived absence of newly acquired cognitive performance skills in a different format leaves the student no option other than use of old response patterns that are ultimately inadequate to the task.

Transitional cognitive behaviors are manifested in hypermobility of thought. When called on for knowledge base responses, the student may appear to sample at random from a professional memory store and not be seeking information in the relevant "section" of the memory bank. These responses may appear to lack even the rudiments of clinical reasoning. In treatment planning, there may be an indication of "throwing" modalities, techniques, assistive devices, and so forth at the task. In particular, occupational therapy students with much background and emphasis on modalities, techniques, and devices as legitimate tools of practice, might resort to these approaches to foster a sense of professionalism. When reporting in team meetings, the inability to identify the most relevant information may result in excess verbiage. Failure to realize the need for prior preparation may contribute to the unmodulated verbal activity.

Mature cognitive behaviors represent a mobility of thought emanating from a stable knowledge base. The student can recognize, understand, and accept the relative lack of competence or knowledge as a natural part of professional development and begin to take corrective action. The student takes the

initiative for seeking information or skill acquisition without the need for attri-
bution of the deficiency to personal inadequacies or to those who have directed
the student's education. When reporting information, the student is able to organize information, select that which is most relevant, and present the information
in a relatively succinct manner.

Psychosocial System

The psychosocial system is called on when the student must deal with interpersonal issues involving clients, family members, or staff members. The *primitive
responses* invoked for ego defense can involve projection to the patient ("That
patient is crazy; nobody can talk to him," "She is so unmotivated," etc.). If the
challenge is for interaction with a staff member, avoidance of interaction can be
present. *Derogation* of the staff member can convey that there is no need for
interaction by the student. These are behaviors that tend to obviate the need for
interaction. Thus, there is no requirement for movement on the student's part
from current perceptions of the person or persons who would be participants in
interpersonal events. Instead of psychosocial movement, hyperstabilization in
psychosocial behaviors is seen.

Transitional psychosocial behaviors, characterized by hypermobility, are
typified by behaviors involving high-energy interactions without adequate regu-
lation. When interacting with patients, students may engage in the "talking"
therapy in an attempt to get the patient moving. "Don't you want to get better?"
"Cheer up. You think you have it bad, look at that patient over there." In an
effort to interact with staff members as "one of the group" instead of the reti-
cence seen with the primitive behaviors, there may be an extreme opposite
reaction. Enthusiasm that intrudes on the personal space of staff members
(both literally and figuratively) indicates psychosocial mobility without the mod-
erating effects of modulating stability.

The student responding with *mature behaviors* is more likely to listen to
the feeling content of patient objections and address the patient at that level.
Another requirement, which is often difficult for the student, involves appropriate confrontation and limit setting. Rather than trying to talk the patient into
improving, the task demands are graded and structured to facilitate activity and
patient progress. In dealing with staff member interactions, the student who
enters fieldwork with an awareness of the need for sensitivity to facility-specific
social and cultural norms will more likely find interpersonal interactions a positive experience and an inducement to professional development.

Suggestions for the Fieldwork Educator and Student

The model of student transition presented in this article is intended to offer a
description of a professional transition as it is manifested in behavior. The model

is intended to describe behaviors rather than prescribe interventions for the supervisor. However, there are implications for both the educator and the student.

For the fieldwork educator, it is important to recognize that student performance in fieldwork is characterized by variability. The educator wants the student to accurately perceive facility expectations and maximize use of personal capabilities to meet those expectations. Frequently, there will be a good fit between facility expectations and student capabilities; at other times, this is not the case. Furthermore, a student may be performing well and exhibiting a predominance of mature behaviors as described in this article. That same student may suddenly exhibit a return to primitive behaviors. This behavior change can signal to the supervisor that the student is feeling somewhat overwhelmed. If the supervisor can recognize this as a normal response, then skillful and sensitive intervention on the supervisor's part can facilitate the student moving away from the primitive behaviors. Without a skillful and sensitive intervention by the supervisor, the student may remain "stuck" in primitive behaviors for a longer period than is necessary or desirable. With effective intervention, the student is relieved of distress with an unsatisfactory performance, views it as normal, and moves on.

It is helpful for the supervisor to remember that throughout fieldwork the student may not move directly to mature behaviors but may exhibit transitional or hypermobile behaviors. Once again, if the supervisor can view this use of transitional behaviors as normative, the supervisor can facilitate a more rapid movement to more mature adaptive response behaviors. It may be necessary to modify facility expectations temporarily—if that is an option. Obviously, with such issues as client safety, expectations cannot be compromised; however, there may be other areas where some temporary relief can be afforded the student.

For students, it is helpful to recognize that there may be variability in their performance, and at times they may experience a sense of not being able to meet facility expectations. Just as the supervisor is encouraged to recognize the expression of primitive behaviors under this circumstance as normal, the student is encouraged to recognize the same. The ability to name and frame their own behaviors can allow students to facilitate their own adaptive movement and act as their own agent of adaptive change. When they cannot engage in self-monitoring and self-correcting actions, then the supervisor's role becomes critical. The most desirable outcome is self-correction on the part of the student, and the active engagement of the student in the corrective process is essential if this goal is to be realized.

For both fieldwork educator and student, the most important factor in using this model of student transition is to recognize performance variations as normative. This realization can relieve supervisors of concerns regarding their role as supervisor, relieve students of the belief that their performance must be error free, and promote dialogue during the supervisory process that enhances the professional performance of both parties.

Research on the Model

To date, there has been one published research study that used the OA model of student transition. Garrett and Schkade (1995) reported a study in which supervisors rated 8 students for whom they had responsibility on a weekly basis. Before the study, supervisors were asked to describe student behaviors relative to facility expectations. A log that the supervisors could use to rate the students was the result of these discussions. The log contained examples of primitive, transitional, and mature behaviors as classified by the researchers. The classes of behavior appeared randomly on the log sheet so as not to induce supervisor rating bias. At the end of 12 weeks, the supervisor ratings were graphed. The graphs reflected predictions made by the model presented herein (i.e., that all three classes of behavior remained in the student's repertoire and that increases in primitive and transitional behaviors appeared in times of particularly stressful challenges). It is important to note that all 8 students performed well, yet there was considerable variability in their individual behavior patterns. The eight graphs appeared in Garrett and Schkade (1995), as did an example from the rating log. One striking case was that in which the student was moved to a different location within the facility halfway into the fieldwork placement. The new unit functioned so differently from the first that there was initially a dramatic increase in primitive and transitional behaviors and a decrease in mature behaviors. Rapidly, however, the student's performance reached previous high levels of mature responses.

The behaviors in the log described in Garrett and Schkade (1995) were specific to the particular facility where the study was conducted. McDonald (1994) converted these behavior descriptions to a more general case and conducted an expert validity study. Fifteen experienced student supervisors were asked to identify the classes of behavior. The log was revised on the basis of the results. Work is currently in progress to see if this log can be used as an approach to communication between supervisor and student and as a counseling tool for the supervisor. Interested fieldwork educators can request a copy of this revised log from the author of this article.

Summary and Conclusions

This article presents a model of student to practitioner on the basis of OA (Schkade & Schultz, 1992; Schultz & Schkade, 1992). Fieldwork supervisors may use this model to think about, communicate about, and facilitate the student developmental process with its inherent undulations. Students may find this model useful in understanding their own responses in fieldwork settings, particularly when the challenges seem overwhelming. This model has the potential to serve as a basis for supervisor–student communication, particularly when a student experiences difficulty. However, it represents only one theoretical approach to fieldwork education. Other educators, both academic and fieldwork, are encouraged to engage in more theory development and testing of theoretical approaches to fieldwork education. Our field has many outstanding fieldwork educators whose knowledge and expertise can be systematized into theoretical frameworks to guide fieldwork education. The art and science of directing fieldwork education can only be enhanced by such efforts. ■

References

Cohn, E. S. (1993). Fieldwork education: Professional socialization. In H. L. Hopkins & H. D. Smith (Eds.), *Willard and Spackman's occupational therapy* (8th ed., pp. 12–19). Philadelphia: Lippincott.

Cohn, E. S., & Crist, P. (1995). Back to the future: New approaches to fieldwork education. *American Journal of Occupational Therapy, 49,* 103–106.

Garrett, S. A., & Schkade, J. K. (1995). Occupational adaptation model of professional development as applied to Level II fieldwork. *American Journal of Occupational Therapy, 49*, 119–126.

Gilfoyle, E. M., Grady, A. P., & Moore, J. C. (1990). *Children adapt* (2nd ed.). Thorofare, NJ: Slack.

Kramer, P., & Stern, K. (1995). Approaches to improving student performance on fieldwork. *American Journal of Occupational Therapy, 49,* 156–159.

McDonald, K. (1994). *Facilitating more effective communication in Level II fieldwork experiences: A counseling tool based on occupational adaptation.* Unpublished manuscript, Texas Woman's University, Denton, TX.

Schkade, J. K. (1991). *Occupational adaptation as a model of professional development: Transition from student to clinician.* Unpublished manuscript.

Schkade, J. K., & Schultz, S. (1992). Occupational adaptation: Toward a holistic approach for contemporary practice: Part 1. *American Journal of Occupational Therapy, 46*, 829–837.

Schon, D. A. (1983). *The reflective practitioner.* New York: Basic Books.

Schultz, S., & Schkade, J. K. (1992). Occupational adaptation: Toward a holistic approach for contemporary practice: Part 2. *American Journal of Occupational Therapy, 46,* 917–925.

Wiemer, R. (1991). Student transition from academic to fieldwork settings. In *Guide to fieldwork education* (pp. 227–233). Rockville, MD: American Occupational Therapy Association.

Differences Between Clinical Reasoning Gainers and Decliners During Fieldwork

Karen Sladyk

Barry G. Sheckley

Karen Sladyk, PhD, OTR/L, FAOTA, is Associate Professor of Occupational Therapy, Bay Path College, Longmeadow, Massachusetts. At the time of this study, she was Assistant Professor of Occupational Therapy, Quinnipiac College, Hamden, Connecticut.

Barry G. Sheckley, PhD, is Professor of Adult and Vocational Education, Department of Educational Leadership, University of Connecticut, Storrs, Connecticut.

Partial funding of this research was provided by the American Occupational Therapy Foundation. The first author is thankful for this support. The study was completed in partial fulfillment of the first author's requirements for a doctoral degree in adult and vocational education at the University of Connecticut.

Objective. Research has supported Level II fieldwork as an effective method of clinical reasoning skill development in students; however, some students benefited more than others. To explain this discrepancy, a study question was developed to examine the perceived differences of the fieldwork experience between high gainers and high decliners on the Clinical Reasoning Case Analysis Test.

Method. Data (N = 70 students) were collected with a researcher-developed case analysis pre- and posttest. Ten students with the highest gains (gainers) and 8 students with the highest declines (decliners) between the pre- and posttests agreed to participate in a semistructured interview after their fieldwork experience. Analysis of themes and frequency counts were used to analyze the interview data to establish which fieldwork experiences helped students develop clinical reasoning skills.

Results. Reflective dialogue activities such as patient interaction, interacting with other fieldwork students beyond treatment issues, and watching other practitioners were highly reported by the students with gains in clinical reasoning as effective in helping the students to think like occupational therapy practitioners. Environmental interferences, such as office politics, were reported as hindering. Getting to know the patient beyond the treatment issues was reported to be the most powerful experience of fieldwork. A model for fieldwork program development is presented.

A SURVEY OF THE LITERATURE SHOWS THAT FIELDWORK HAS had an integral role in occupational therapy education throughout its history (Nystrom, 1986). Although the process and content of fieldwork has been debated over the years, the value of the fieldwork experience to integrate academic knowledge with practice has always been considered important (Pressler, 1983).

Cohn and Frum (1988) stated that developing competent clinical reasoning skills in students is complicated by a rapidly changing clinical environment focused on cost containment, funding, and complex health care technology. Cohn (1989) reported that the need to teach students to examine their practice critically was further complicated by the need for students to learn routine clinical skills during fieldwork. The shortage of occupational therapy practitioners and the demand for high-quality care has led occupational therapy fieldwork educators to insist that both students and new staff members have clinical reasoning skills in addition to technical skills (Cortellini-Benamy, 1990). Fieldwork has been effective in developing clinical reasoning skills in students (Sladyk, 1997), but students who focus only on the development of routine clinical skills during fieldwork will find themselves ill prepared for current practice (Cohn, 1989).

Organizing the learning environment to increase students' clinical reasoning is the responsibility of fieldwork educators (Christie & Cohn, 1989; Joyce & Moeller, 1985). According to Cohn and Frum (1988), not all fieldwork educators are fully prepared. In a field in which fieldwork educators are faced with the complex situation of developing competent occupational therapy practitioners, the problem is how to best facilitate and promote the development of clinical reasoning skills and a reflective stance toward practice in students during fieldwork. As a first step in addressing this dilemma, this study explored the perceived differences in the fieldwork experience between students with high gains and students with high declines in clinical reasoning scores during fieldwork.

Literature Review

Given the responsibility facing clinical supervisors, a model is needed to assist them in understanding the development of clinical reasoning skills in fieldwork students. Theory and research in the fields of adult learning and occupational therapy can contribute to this model by explaining clinical reasoning skill development through experience and reflection.

Clinical Reasoning

An important professional competence in occupational therapy is clinical reasoning. Mattingly and Fleming (1994) presented groundbreaking research in their model of clinical reasoning. Mattingly (1991) noted that clinical reasoning was largely tacit, highly imagistic, and deeply phenomenological in thinking. Fleming (1991) presented clinical reasoning as thinking in three tracks.

1. Procedural
2. Interactive
3. Conditional

Procedural thinking involves the practitioner addressing the diagnosis and the treatment techniques. Interactive thinking involves the practitioner and patient communicating with each other. Conditional thinking involves the practitioner viewing patients within the context of the patient's own environment. According to Fleming (1991), expert occupational therapy practitioners use all three tracks of clinical reasoning in the smooth integration of treatment. As expert occupational therapy practitioners develop clinical reasoning through their experiences, experiential learning models may assist the novice fieldwork student to begin to develop clinical reasoning skills.

Learning From Experience

From Dewey's (1938) classic work and related research, Kolb (1984) developed a formulation of experiential learning theory (ELT). Kolb described learning as a process in which constructed knowledge resulted from the transformation of experience. Because fieldwork involves the development of professional knowledge through experience with occupational therapy consumers, Kolb's model of understanding learning from experience can help explain the development of clinical reasoning skills in students. ELT involves transforming experiences into knowledge with reflection and experimentation. Because fieldwork inherently involves experimentation, the role of reflection was of particular interest to this study.

Reflection has been discussed by many (Buermeyer et al., 1923; Canning, 1991; Kolb, 1984; Osterman, 1990; Schon, 1983; Sheckley & Keeton, 1997; Sparks-Langer & Colton, 1991). Although difficult to operationalize due to its complexity, reflection has been studied in both qualitative and quantitative research. Qualitative research by Canning (1991) and Policinski and Davidhizar (1985) showed that the idea of reflection can cause ambivalence and confusion in students when old ideas of the learner are challenged. Hollingsworth (1990) found that, until new teachers mastered everyday management of the classroom, the teachers were unable to be reflective about student outcomes. Lampert and Clark (1990) found that reflective teachers monitored both cognitive thinking and the effects of their actions. Berkey and associates (1990) found that reflective activities were more meaningful to and more effective for professional teachers when the teachers chose the activities themselves and the school provided release time to participate.

Quantitative research in reflection showed promise for further investigation in occupational therapy. Studies with large effect sizes (statistical analysis explaining a large variance as well as a statistical probability) were of interest to the authors. Two studies showed large effect sizes (Carpenter, Fennema, Peterson, Chiang, & Loef, 1989; Sparks-Langer, Simmons, Pasch, Colton, & Starko, 1990). Carpenter et al. (1989) found that teachers in graduate studies who were exposed to research about teaching reading but were not instructed in how to use the techniques, nonetheless, incorporated the research into their teaching. Sparks-Langer and colleagues (1990) showed that student teachers in a reflective fieldwork environment performed much higher than students in a traditional fieldwork program. Further research combining reflection and clinical reasoning skills could assist occupational therapy students in meeting the demands of practice.

Purpose of This Study

Earlier research (Sladyk, 1997) showed that fieldwork develops clinical reasoning in students ($p < 0.01$, large effect size) as measured by the Clinical Reasoning Case Analysis Test (CRCAT) developed by Sladyk (1997); however, some students benefited more than others. To begin to address the issues of developing an effective fieldwork model to develop clinical reasoning skills in students, the following research question was developed: In what ways do fieldwork students with the greatest increases and decreases on the CRCAT agree and differ in their perceptions about how various fieldwork activities contributed to their learning occupational therapy?

Method

Sample

As part of a larger quantitative study ($N = 70$) on clinical reasoning and field-work (Sladyk, 1997), students completed pre- and posttest case studies to measure their clinical reasoning in procedural, interactive, and conditional thinking. The CRCAT was developed by the first author and used an agreement index of 0.98 for validity. Cronbach's α of 0.87 established reliability. Seventy percent of students gained on the posttest (gainers), whereas 30% declined on the posttest (decliners).

In this study, 22 fieldwork students with the greatest changes in CRCAT pre- and posttest scores were asked to participate in an interview, conducted by the first author, concerning their perception of activities used in fieldwork. Ten gainers and 8 decliners agreed to be interviewed and participated fully. Eighteen persons allowed for data saturation, and no further interviews were conducted. Interviewees reflected the type of fieldwork assignments for the original sample with 11 (65%) on their first fieldwork placement for mental health and 7 participants (37%) on their second fieldwork placement for physical management.

Data Collection

By using a semistructured format, the first author asked students about experiences in fieldwork that were helpful or hindered their thinking like an occupational therapy practitioner. They were further asked about the role of reflection during fieldwork. Interviews were completed 6 to 8 weeks after the completion of the fieldwork experience.

In the interview session, participants were allowed to answer the questions in their own way, without particular definitions from the interviewer. Interviews were face to face if the student was available but were mainly conducted on the telephone because most students lived out of state. To avoid bias, interviewees were not told they had been selected because of their scores on the CRCAT or what scores they had received but were simply told their name had been selected as part of a follow-up to the survey they had completed earlier. Because the interviewer was aware of the interviewees' scores, both gainers and decliners were asked the same questions. All interviews were tape recorded and transcribed for analysis.

Data Analysis

Interview data were analyzed by using methods to develop codes and themes from the interview and analyzing frequency of responses within themes (Lincoln

& Guba, 1985; Marshall & Rossman, 1995). Themes are described below. Raw data and thematic analyses were audited by an experienced ELT researcher to determine whether the conclusions were reasonable.

Results

Surprisingly, interviewees with gaining scores on the CRCAT had a mean grade point average (GPA) of 3.29, and interviewees with declining scores on the CRCAT had a mean GPA of 3.46. An independent t test showed there were no significant differences in GPA between gainers and decliners ($t = -1.0$, $p = 0.89$), and both gainers and decliners were similar to the overall sample GPA of 3.33.

Interviewees were asked how important they believed fieldwork was in helping them to think like an occupational therapy practitioner. Twelve participants believed that fieldwork was very important, and only one believed it was not important. Because saturation was reached, and no pattern of answers were found in gaining and declining scorers, the question was not asked of everyone. The results were expected because most students believe that fieldwork is an important aspect of their education.

Interviewees were next asked to give three examples of fieldwork activities that helped them to think like an occupational therapy practitioner. Students most commonly reported patient-related treatments or interactions with patients as helpful. When explaining themselves, the students often told a story about a particular patient. Often the story was more detailed than merely citing medical information, a characteristic that demonstrated that students were using clinical reasoning skills beyond those characteristics of the procedural track to include characteristics of interactive and conditional reasoning (Mattingly & Fleming, 1994).

Gaining scorers were more likely to include interactive and conditional details in their patient stories versus the stories of students who lost points on the CRCAT posttest. Specifically, gaining scorers identified the importance of getting to know the patient through conversation (interactive reasoning) and viewed the patient as a person within the person's environment (conditional reasoning). For example, a student who had gained 40 points on the CRCAT said:

> One thing that happened on fieldwork was a patient who only spoke Spanish. There wasn't a single person on staff who spoke Spanish but me. I was the only person who could interact with him. He came over [from Puerto Rico to the United States], leaving his pregnant wife at home. He lived with the rest of his family to make money. He was in a manic phase but no one could understand what was in this poor person's head. I just tried to interact with him a little bit. He ignored the rest of the staff unless he saw me coming, then he would smile. Staff would get upset with him because when he had visitors, the whole family would visit, they would be crying, it would disturb the whole unit. Dealing with him made me think of the patient as a person, not a diagnosis.

Other students who lost points on the CRCAT posttest had similar patient stories. Although not as detailed as the student above and more focused on procedural reasoning, a student who declined by 36 points on the CRCAT posttest indicated the ways in which fieldwork promoted the development of clinical reasoning skills.

> I also did a high motor activity for a lady [with profound mental retardation] whose joints were not all that good. It was really cool. She could not speak either. And just understanding where she was coming from, I really learnt [sic] tolerance [in carrying out procedures]. To know when to push and when not to.

Students next reported three program characteristics most often in discussing activities that helped them think like an occupational therapy practitioner. These included having other students with them ($n = 6$), being able to watch other practitioners during treatment ($n = 9$), and getting feedback from their supervisor ($n = 6$). Gainers on the CRCAT were 5 times more likely to report the benefits of having other students with them ($n = 5$) and twice as likely to report being able to watch other practitioners during treatment ($n = 6$) compared with their peers who declined on the clinical reasoning test. Gaining scorers and declining scorers on the CRCAT were even in reporting the benefit of supervisor feedback.

One student who gained 44 points between the pre- and post-CRCAT demonstrated the importance of having another student with her to develop her clinical reasoning skills.

> There was another student from USC. We could blow off steam with each other and bounce ideas off each other. There were a lot of OTs, over 12 OTs and OTAs and a large treatment area, so I got to watch a lot of treatments.

Several additional themes were present in the activities students stated were important in helping them think like an occupational therapy practitioner. One was the importance of developing a professional sense of self. This theme was evident when students reported the benefits of just watching other practitioners or getting feedback from the supervisor. Second, students seemed to value the quality of the experiences over the quantity of the experiences. This seemed particularly true in the patient interaction stories. Students seemed to value having time to really get to know their patients.

Because the purpose of fieldwork is to develop clinical reasoning skills and apply the reflective stance to practice (AOTA, 1991), the type of activities that led to the development of clinical reasoning skills in students were of particular interest to this study. ELTs were found to provide a framework that embraced the learning-from-experience themes of the fieldwork activities reported by the participants. Results are presented in Table 1.

Activities that promote reflection were most frequently reported ($n = 52$). Dialogue activities were the highest reported subcategory of activities that

Table 1
Activities That Interviewees Perceived Helped Them To Think Like an Occupational Therapy Practitioner by Gaining and Declining Scores on the CRCAT

Activities	Total	Gaining	Declining
Dialogue Activities	32	21	11
Patient interaction, other students with me, talk or watch other practitioners, feedback from supervisor, control or responsibility for my own learning, mixing mental health with physical management, journal writing, supervisor was role model, patients who did not get better			
Action Activities	20	7	13
Patient treatment, used freedom to be creative or experiment, made a project, documented, covered for my supervisor			
Working With Others	7	4	3
Attended team meeting, different supervisors, structured student program, intense case load			
Academic Assignments	4	3	1
Conducted an in-service presentation			

helped interviewees develop clinical reasoning. Thirty-two activities were reported in this subcategory, more than all the other categories combined. Gaining scorers were nearly twice as likely to report dialogue activities as their peers with declining scores on the CRCAT. Action activities were reported second to reflective dialogue with 20 total experiences. Working with and observing professionals was reported seven times. Gaining scorers and declining scorers were almost evenly split when describing experiences working with professionals that helped to develop clinical reasoning. Academic assignments were reported the least, with only four total experiences noted, and all of these students conducted in-service presentations.

In contrast to activities that helped students to think like an occupational therapy practitioner, interviewees were asked what activities they participated in that did not help, that hindered them, or were a waste of time. In this case, interviewees described a broader scope of activities, events, and attitudes rather than specific activities. Examples included staff member conflicts, blurred boundaries, Joint Commission on Accreditation of Healthcare Organizations visits, occupational therapy not respected, lack of resources, patients did not get better, and being the sole student. These were often outside environmental factors versus activities in which the student participated. Kolb (1984) referred to these as *environmental presses*. Of the environmental interference reported, only "staff had conflicts" and "blurred professional boundaries" were reported by more than 3 interviewees.

Interviewees, despite whether they were gaining or declining scorers, were three times more likely to report an environmental interference versus other activities as a hindering factor in their thinking like an occupational therapy practitioner. One student who declined by 36 points on the CRCAT discussed the effect of too much control from the supervisor.

> There was a lot of conflict between the therapies, which made things difficult at times. The supervisor was all for me as the student, and she didn't want me to get stuck in the middle, but sometimes she took that too far. She would be too protective.

As a result, the student believed that her clinical reasoning skills were hindered.

When specifically looking at student activities, interviewees reported that academic assignments did not help them think like an occupational therapy practitioner. This is not surprising because these assignments are similar to classroom activities, and students want to be more active on fieldwork. One student who gained 42 points on the CRCAT demonstrated her lack of interest in academic assignments.

> My supervisor made us research a topic she was working on. I had no interest in it, and I thought it was a waste of time.

Interviewees were further asked to describe their most powerful experience during fieldwork. As with the question of three activities that helped the interviewee think like an occupational therapy practitioner, the most powerful experiences were ones that promoted reflective dialogue. The most common answer was some type of patient interaction, with 9 interviewees stating this as the most powerful. No other answer received more than two responses. Key to the interviewees was the importance of dialogue that triggered reflection on the effect of therapeutic use of self and the effectiveness of interactive reasoning. One student who gained 44 points on the CRCAT said:

> Albert H. was an above-knee amputee. He was so nasty when he got there [in rehabilitation], but he connected with me because I was the same age as a daughter he had lost. He was just so grumpy. When he left, he and his wife gave me roses.

This indicates the student's therapeutic use of self in the interactive track of clinical reasoning. Last, students were asked if fieldwork made them more reflective and when reflection started. Almost all the gainers (90%) stated that fieldwork made them more reflective. Of the interviewees who declined on the clinical reasoning test, 63% were still likely to report fieldwork as making them more reflective. Typical of those who said fieldwork made them more reflective was this interviewee who gained 50 points on the CRCAT.

> I was more reflective by the end. When I first went in, I just took things as they were. Then I could think things through, like why did a patient do this? Why did they act out this way?

This quote indicates the change in the student from a person who just accepted the situation to someone who questioned the possibilities.

All interviewees, despite whether they believed that fieldwork made them more reflective or if reflection remained the same, were asked when reflection on fieldwork began for them. Forty-four percent of the interviewees believed reflection began at the end of fieldwork. Of interest is that no interviewees said they were reflective from the beginning of fieldwork. Being consciously aware of reflection typically came at the end of the fieldwork or after. This is likely due to the nature of the busy clinical setting. Students may not have a chance to "catch their breath" and realize that a change was occurring in their practice. Typical of the responses on the start of reflection was this interviewee who declined by 36 points on the CRCAT: "During the actual affiliation, it was just get things done." This statement seemed to highlight the procedural component of clinical reasoning and underscore the task (as opposed to reflective) nature of the fieldwork setting.

Discussion

This investigation took the first step in identifying factors that affect the development of clinical reasoning skills and a reflective stance toward practice in fieldwork students. Relationships between activities thought to develop clinical reasoning skills in fieldwork students (Cohn, 1989) and changes seen in fieldwork students showed little correlation. Further investigation showed the importance of reflective dialogue activities in the process of learning how to think like an occupational therapy practitioner. For example, the importance of developing a relationship with the patient beyond the treatment aspects, the importance of watching other professionals, and the effect of having other students with them during fieldwork was articulated often by students who gained on the CRCAT. The quality of the fieldwork experiences versus the quantity of the experiences was likewise articulated.

Sheckley and Keeton (1997) argued that experience is actively constructed and that the experience is the vehicle that promotes "deep processing" of information. Over time, cognitive processing becomes automatic when experience matches the person's schema. Bandura (1993) supported this automated view of experience processing, noting that repetition of a task requires little attention or cognitive resources. The effect of this automatization is the removal of the reflective process from the experiential learning cycle (Sheckley & Keeton, 1997). Surprises can disrupt the automatization effect of the learning cycle. When this occurs, the learning cycle then expands outward, like an accordion (Sheckley & Keeton, 1997). The process engages an episodic memory process in a way that results in permanent restructuring of knowledge. By following the expanded model of experiential learning of Sheckley and Keeton (1997), effective occupational therapy fieldwork programs would not only develop population-specific technical skills in students that would promote "automatic" responses to specific patient symptoms, but also they would use "experiential surprises" to assist students in developing reflective flexibility skills that would enable them to deeply process the information and be able to transfer it to use with different populations. These experiential surprises seemed to come from reflective dialogue activities such as the importance of developing a relationship with the patient beyond the treatment aspects, the importance of watching other professionals, and the effect of having other students with them during fieldwork.

Implications for Fieldwork Supervision

A model to encourage reflective dialogue activities as an integrated part of fieldwork is presented in Figure 1. The role of dialogue activities acts as an accordion to expand out the richness of the fieldwork experience. Fieldwork supervisors may want to consider dropping traditional fieldwork assignments such as case studies and conducting an in-service presentation in favor of opportunities to dialogue with the student. These opportunities should not be formal or structured like planned supervision; rather, they should be time when a student can talk with or watch other professionals in action. The supervising occupational therapy practitioner can used planned supervision time to assist the student in linking experiences he or she has had.

Limitations

As stated before, this study is just the first step in exploring how fieldwork students develop clinical reasoning. The authors acknowledge that several limitations exist, such as selection bias in the convenient volunteer population; however, the sample was typical of occupational therapy students nationwide in age and gender. The 3 months between the pre- and posttests used to establish the gainers and decliners may have provided other experiences not studied and is accepted as a limitation. Furthermore, details about the students' experiences, such as time spent with consumers, were not addressed. Results are delimited to the sample of Level II fieldwork students from a small, private college in New England. The degree to which the results can be generalized is dependent on the degree to which similarities exist between the group studied and other samples.

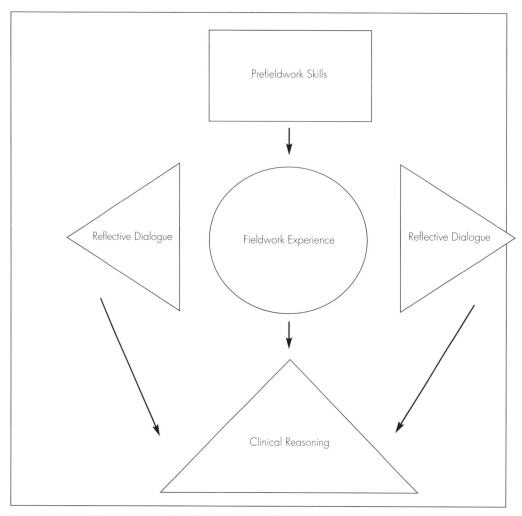

Figure 1. Model to improve clinical reasoning skills.

Future Research

The results and conclusions of this study continue to raise many questions regarding the development of clinical reasoning skills and a reflective stance to practice in Level II fieldwork students, including

■ What role do parallel nonclinical processes, such as learning to manage the political nature of the workplace, have on the development of clinical reasoning skills?

■ Are there any other differences between those learners who gain clinical reasoning skills on fieldwork and those who decline? Do decliners ever catch up to gainers? How does more experience affect decliners?

■ How do fieldwork programs that focus on reflective dialogue activities differ from fieldwork programs that use a more eclectic approach? Does type of fieldwork (e.g., mental health or physical management) affect the level of reflective dialogue activities used? ■

References

American Occupational Therapy Association. (1991). *Commission on education: Guide to fieldwork education.* Bethesda, MD: Author.

Bandura, A. (1993). Perceived self-efficacy in cognitive development and functioning. *Educational Psychologist, 28*(2), 117–148.

Berkey, R., Curtis, T., Minnick, F., Zietlow, K., Campbell, D., & Kirschner, B. (1990). Collaborating for reflective practice. *Education and Urban Society, 22*, 204–232.

Buermeyer, L., Cooley, W. F., Coss, J. J., Friess, H. L., Gutmann, J., Munro, T., Peterson, H., Randall, J. H., & Schneider, H. W. (1923). *An introduction to reflective thinking.* Boston: Houghton Mifflin.

Canning, C. (1991). What teachers say about reflection. *Educational Leadership, 48*, 18–21.

Carpenter, T. P., Fennema, E., Peterson, P. L., Chiang, C., & Loef, M. (1989). Using knowledge of children's mathematics thinking in classroom teaching: An experimental study. *American Educational Research Journal, 26*, 499–531.

Christie, B., Joyce, P., & Moeller, P. (1985). Fieldwork experience: Impact on practice preference. *American Journal of Occupational Therapy, 39*, 671–674.

Cohn, E. S. (1989). Fieldwork education: Shaping a foundation for clinical reasoning. *American Journal of Occupational Therapy, 43*, 240–244.

Cohn, E. S. & Frum, D. (1988). The Issue Is—Fieldwork supervision: More education is warranted. *American Journal of Occupational Therapy, 42*, 325–327.

Cortellini-Benamy, B. (1990). Clinical reasoning, entry level therapists and students. *Administration and Management Special Interest Section Newsletter, 6*(2), 1–3.

Dewey, J. (1938). *Experience in education.* New York: Collier.

Fleming, M. (1991). The therapist with the three track mind. *American Journal of Occupational Therapy, 45*, 1007–1014.

Hollingsworth, S. (1990, April 17).*Teacher educator as researcher: An epistemological analysis of learning to teach reading.* Paper presented at the annual meeting of the American Educational Research Association, Boston, MA.

Kolb, D. (1984). *Experiential learning.* Englewood Cliffs, NJ: Prentice-Hall.

Lampert, M., & Clark, C. M. (1990). Expert knowledge and expert thinking in teaching: A response to Floden and Klinzing. *Educational Researcher, 19*(4), 21–23.

Lincoln, Y., & Guba, E. (1985). *Naturalistic inquiry.* Beverly Hills, CA: Sage.

Marshall, C., & Rossman, G. B. (1995). *Designing qualitative research.* Beverly Hills, CA: Sage.

Mattingly, C. (1991). What is clinical reasoning? *American Journal of Occupational Therapy, 45,* 979–986.

Mattingly, C., & Fleming, M. (1994). *Clinical reasoning.* Philadelphia: F. A. Davis.

Nystrom, E. P. (1986). The differentiation between academic and fieldwork education. In *Occupational therapy education: Target 2000 proceedings* (pp. 90–94). Bethesda, MD: American Occupational Therapy Association.

Osterman, K. (1990). Reflective practice: A new agenda for education. *Education and Urban Society, 22,* 133–152.

Policinski, H., & Davidhizar, R. (1985). Mentoring the novice. *Nurse Educator, 10*(3), 34–37.

Presseler, S. (1983). Fieldwork education, the proving ground of the profession. *American Journal of Occupational Therapy, 37,* 163–165.

Schon, D. (1983). *The reflective practitioner: How professionals think in action.* New York: Basic Books.

Sheckley, B., & Keeton, M. (1997). *Perspectives on how adults learn: A framework for discussing approaches to workforce development.* Paper presented to Council for Adult and Experiential Learning Board of Trustees, San Diego, CA.

Sladyk, K. (1997). *Clinical reasoning and reflective practice: Influence of fieldwork activities.* Unpublished doctoral dissertation, University of Connecticut, Storrs.

Sparks-Langer, G. M., & Colton, A. B. (1991). Synthesis of research on teachers' reflective thinking. *Educational Leadership, 48,* 37–44.

Sparks-Langer, G. M., Simmons, J. M., Pasch, M., Colton, A. B., & Starko, A. (1990). Reflective pedagogical thinking: How can we promote it and measure it? *Journal of Teacher Education, 41,* 23–32.

Should the Clinical Doctorate Degree Be the Standard of Entry Into the Practice of Occupational Therapy?

Charlotte Brasic Royeen

Sidney J. Stohs

Charlotte Brasic Royeen, PhD, OTR, FAOTA, is Chairperson, Education Special Interest Section, American Occupational Therapy Association, and Associate Dean for Research and Professor in Occupational Therapy, School of Pharmacy and Allied Health Professions, Creighton University, Omaha, Nebraska.

Sidney J. Stohs, PhD, is Dean, School of Pharmacy and Allied Health Professions, Creighton University, Omaha, Nebraska.

This essay briefly addresses key issues surrounding the clinical doctorate degree for occupational therapy. Given the general lack of knowledge about this degree and its function, this article provides the reader with basic information on the clinical doctorate. In doing so, our goal is to provide an entree for scholarly debate on the relative merits of this degree for entry-level education in occupational therapy. Considering societal needs and the demands of professional practice, it is our fervent belief that the clinical doctorate is the most appropriate degree for entry-level education in occupational therapy. A series of 10 question-and-answer summaries follow and present our view of the clinical doctorate.

What Is the Clinical Doctorate in Occupational Therapy?

The clinical doctorate is not a new degree per se, but it is a new degree for the field of occupational therapy. The clinical doctorate is a professional degree. It is not a graduate school degree. The clinical doctorate may be considered a clinical degree (like the master of occupational therapy [MOT]) but not an academic degree (like the master of science in occupational therapy [MSOT]). It is a practice-based, clinical degree. The reader is referred to other sources for more information on the history of the clinical doctorate (Pierce & Peyton, in press) as well as for a framework for developing a clinical doctorate in a university (Threlkeld, Jensen, & Royeen, in press).

How Is a Clinical Doctorate Different From Other Doctorates in Occupational Therapy?

The standard and familiar doctoral program in occupational therapy is the doctor of philosophy (PhD) degree, which is a graduate, research-based, academic degree that differs from clinical doctorates, which are clinically focused professional degrees. Generally speaking, the PhD educates the student in traditional scholarship (i.e., the processes of discovery of knowledge as well as theory development). The clinical doctorate educates the student in the application and synthesis of theory and practice-based knowledge, which is a more recently recognized area of scholarship (Glassick, Huber, & Maeroff, 1997).

How Did the Clinical Doctorate in Occupational Therapy Come To Exist?

Professional competence and professional attitudes resulting in professional performance outcomes at the level society requires are concepts discussed by Stark, Lowther, Hagarty, and Orcyk (1986) in terms of development of a profession. The level of professional performance outcomes demanded of occupational therapy practitioners as they move into more nontraditional practice settings is consistent with education at the level of the clinical doctorate. Indeed, it can be argued that, for many years, occupational therapy has awarded the "wrong degree" for the work scope and performance outcomes associated with the education. For example, the first author received a baccalaureate degree for a level of work for which other professions granted a master's degree. Seminal articles by Rogers (1980a, 1980b) addressed the morass of degree structures that occupational therapy was implementing outside of traditional academic structures. We believe that implementation of the clinical doctorate, similar to the clinical doctorates in medicine (MD) or and dentistry (DDS), fits with existing university structure and policies. In fact, to be consistent with the degree developments that have occurred in other health care professions, the establishment of the clinical doctorate is a natural and logical progression.

How Does the Clinical Doctorate in Occupational Therapy Compare With Clinical Doctorates in Other Fields?

This has already been briefly discussed; however, it is important to emphasize how the clinical doctorate is consistent with education in other professions. The clinical doctorate is structured in a manner consistent with the structure of clinical dictates in the other health professions (Runyon, Aitken, & Stohs, 1994). The most commonly recognized model of the clinical doctorate is the aforementioned MD degree, which is characterized by premedical requirements, admission into the program, and a professional didactic curriculum followed by intensive clinical education. In addition to dentistry, other health professions that use this model include pharmacy with the doctor of pharmacy (PharmD) degree and the more recent development in physical therapy of the doctor of physical therapy (DPT) degree. By using the clinical doctorate and the research doctorate as "standards," occupational therapy can avoid problems and confusion that have developed in other fields such as nursing, where four kinds of nursing doctoral programs exist in addition to the research-based PhD program.

Why Is the Clinical Doctorate in Occupational Therapy Important to the Profession?

The clinical doctorate program is important for occupational therapy because it fulfills both societal and professional needs. Among other things, society needs practitioners skilled in communication, interdisciplinary teamwork, clinical reasoning, and cultural sensitivity (Shugars, O'Neil, & Bader, 1991). Professional needs will be met by following a "power" approach most recognized in the literature on development of a profession. Professional power is "power held by practitioners in their social exchange and services to individual clients" (Forsyth & Daniesenicz, 1985, p. 61). It concerns public recognition of the important service the profession provides to society overall. The clinical doctorate allows for use of "Dr." as a form of address. Thus, the degree itself and designation of "Dr." will add to the overall stature and recognition of occupational therapy practitioners in their service to society. The profession of pharmacy has mandated change from baccalaureate-level education to entry level at the clinical doctorate. Thus, there is precedent for a profession making a comprehensive change in level of entry.

Why Is the Clinical Doctorate Important to Consumers of Occupational Therapy Services?

The greater depth and professional education provided by clinical doctorate education is more likely to result in practitioners who meet professional competencies as well as professional attitudes identified by Stark et al. (1986). (It is beyond the scope of this chapter to discuss these competencies. The reader should refer to the original source.) These professional competencies are

- conceptual competence,
- technical competence,
- integrative competence,
- contextual competence,
- adaptive competence, and
- interpersonal communication.

Additionally, the professional attitudes identified by Fidler (1996) are probably best achieved and socialized at the level of clinical doctoral education. They are

- professional identity,
- professional ethics,
- career marketability,
- scholarly concern for improvement, and
- motivation for continued learning.

These outcome competencies from clinical doctorate education result in practitioners who have a greater depth of knowledge and a greater ability to apply knowledge in diverse and nontraditional settings (i.e., the scholarship of integration and application as defined by Glassick et al. [1997]). Furthermore, these practitioners are prepared to more rapidly understand and apply innovation. The net result is that clients and systems will receive a higher and more efficient level of care.

Because There Is a Shortage of Qualified Faculty Members at the PhD Level, How Can Entry at the Clinical Doctorate Level Be Supported?

In the American system of economics, demand influences supply, and supply influences demand. Arguing that we cannot support programs of education at the level of a clinical doctorate means that we will never have the resources to support such an endeavor. It is, in essence, a self-defeating rationale. Movement toward clinical doctorate education would increase the need for faculty members trained at varied doctoral levels, and the need could be effectively used to lobby Congress and other organizations to better fund and attend to the critical shortage of well-qualified faculty members in occupational therapy.

Additionally, although one assumes that the PhD is necessary for optimal faculty status and performance, it should be remembered that the PhD degree is a research degree, whereas the clinical doctorate is just that, namely a degree from programs with a clinical emphasis versus a research emphasis. Educational programs providing the clinical doctorate degree do not require that all faculty members have a PhD. As with medical schools or schools of pharmacy, faculty members usually have a collection of PhD and professional doctorates such as MDs or PharmDs.

Why Would Entry at the Master's Degree Level Be Inadequate for Occupational Therapy Education?

An MOT is not consistent with the degree structures used by the vast majority of health professions. An entry-level professional master's degree adds to the degree confusion in the light of the long-standing acceptance and recognition of the graduate, research-focused MS degrees (Rogers, 1980a, 1980b).

What About the Cost Involved? Will a Clinical Doctorate Cost More?

A clinical doctorate is a more intensive degree and requires a greater time commitment. As a result, the cost of education is higher. As with any professional doctoral program, the costs associated with the educational program may be recouped over time as the result of higher salaries. The salary question, however, is a marketplace issue and is not determined by educational institutions. The clinical doctorate in occupational therapy provides greater employment and advancement opportunities and, therefore, greater reimbursement opportunities.

What Might Happen if Occupational Therapy Does Not Move to Entry Level at the Clinical Doctorate?

In the rapidly changing health care environment, the stature of occupational therapy can be expected to diminish if the profession does not move toward entry level at the clinical doctorate. The field of occupational therapy would likely become a technical-level, paraprofessional field. Occupational therapy education must change to meet the evolving health care delivery system and remain competitive in the health care and human services marketplace.

Summary

It is beyond the scope of this brief essay to provide an in-depth analysis of the rationale for the clinical doctorate to become the level of entry into occupational therapy. In a cursory manner, we have provided the reader with an overview of critical issues surrounding the clinical doctorate. We suggest truncating lengthy scholarly debate on the pros and cons of moving to the clinical doctorate for entry level because, by the time scholarly discourse has been completed, the world will have "moved on." If occupational therapy does not move to the clinical doctorate for entry level, occupational therapy might find itself to be a technical, not professional, field. Thus, we answer the question, "Should the clinical doctorate degree be the standard of entry into the practice of occupational therapy?" with a resounding, "Yes!"

Reilly (1962) suggested that occupational therapy could be one of the great ideas of the 20th century. But within the cacophony of competition as well as the need to respond to societal change, occupational therapy will continue as a profession and be a great idea for the 21st century, only with the designation "Dr." ◼

Acknowledgments

The pioneering work of Claudia Peyton, MS, OTR, Chair, Department of Occupational Therapy, School of Pharmacy and Allied Health Professions, Creighton University (Omaha, NE) in the development of a clinical doctorate is acknowledged, as is the influence of our colleague, Gail M. Jensen, PhD, LPT.

References

Fidler, G. S. (1996). Developing a repertoire of professional behaviors. *American Journal of Occupational Therapy, 50*, 583–587.

Forsyth, P. B., & Danisenicz, T. J. (1985). Towards a theory of professionalization. *Work and Occupations, 12*(1), 59–76.

Glassick, C. E., Huber, M. T., & Maeroff, G. I. (1997). *Scholarship assessed: Evaluation of the professoriate*. San Francisco: Jossey-Bass.

Pierce, D., & Peyton, C. (1999). An historical cross-disciplinary perspective on the clinical doctorate. *American Journal of Occupational Therapy, 53,* 64–71.

Reilly, M. (1962). Occupational therapy can be one of the great ideas of 20th century medicine. *American Journal of Occupational Therapy, 16,* 1–9.

Rogers, J. C. (1980a). Design of the master's degree in occupational therapy. Part 1: A logical approach. *American Journal of Occupational Therapy, 34,* 113–118.

Rogers, J. C. (1980b). Design of the master's degree in occupational therapy. Part 2: An empirical approach. *American Journal of Occupational Therapy, 34,* 176–184.

Runyon, C. P., Aitken, M. J., & Stohs, S. J. (1994, Spring). The need for a clinical doctorate in occupational therapy education. *Journal of Allied Health, 23*(2), 57–63.

Shugars, D. A., O'Neil, E. H., & Bader, J. D. (Eds.). (1991). *Healthy Americans: Practitioners for 2005: An agenda for action for U.S. health professions schools.* Durham, NC: Pew Health Professions Committee.

Stark, J., Lowther, M., Hagarty, B., & Orcyk, C. (1986). A conceptual framework for the study of preservice professional programs in colleges and universities. *Journal of Higher Education, 57,* 231–258.

Threlkeld, A. J., Jensen, G., & Royeen, C. B. (in press). The clinical doctorate: An analysis framework for physical therapy. *Journal of Physical Therapy.*

Information for Authors

The *Innovations in Occupational Therapy Education* (IOTE) Editor invites manuscript submissions that conform to its aim and scope without regard to the professional affiliations of authors. Five types of contributions are considered:

1. Full-length or feature articles
2. Brief reports
3. Letters to the editor
4. Book, monograph, and technology reviews
5. Commentaries

Guidelines for preparing and submitting manuscripts are outlined subsequently. Manuscripts that do not substantially comply with these guidelines will be returned to the author(s) without consideration.

Manuscript Preparation

All manuscripts should be prepared according to the IOTE Requirements for Submission of Manuscripts and Disks.

General Style and Format Considerations

Authors should prepare manuscripts in accordance with the latest (1994) edition of the *Publication Manual of the American Psychological Association* (APA). Neither the American Occupational Therapy Association nor IOTE editorial staff members can assume responsibility for statements or opinions expressed by authors. Authors are strongly encouraged to consult the APA publication manual (4th edition), for more detailed advice on the preparation of manuscripts.

Specific Guidelines by Type of Contribution

Feature Articles

Full-length research articles should generally not exceed 4,000 words (15 double-spaced typewritten pages, including tables, references, and figures). Each article must be accompanied by an abstract that clearly, completely, and succinctly summarizes the material that follows. Abstracts of empirical studies should be 100 to 150 words in length; theoretical articles should be 75 to 100 words. Each article must be accompanied by a one-sentence explanation of how this work will benefit occupational therapy practitioners or the practice of occupational therapy. Pages should be numbered consecutively (except for figures) in the following order: title page (page 1), abstract (page 2), text (beginning on page 3), references (new page after text), appendices (each on a new page), and tables and figures (each on separate pages). This arrangement is necessary for copy processing and does not represent how the manuscript will appear in print. Identify each manuscript page (except the figures) by typing the first 2 to 3 words from the title in the upper right-hand corner above the page number.

The title page should contain the authors' names, affiliations, complete mailing address, e-mail address, and telephone and fax numbers. It should include the one-sentence explanation of the work's relevance to occupational therapy. The title page should list acknowledgments, grant or contract support, and information concerning previous presentation of the material at symposia or conferences.

Briefs

IOTE will publish expanded descriptions of innovative approaches to fieldwork instructional methods and research in education outcomes. Submitted manuscripts in this category must be limited to 1,000 words and be as succinct, accurate, and informative as possible.

Reviews

Book, monograph, journal, and technology reviews are limited to 500 words and should include an objective and substantive appraisal of the item's merit. Provide the names of authors, the title in full, the publisher and city, the date or frequency of publication, the number of pages, and the purchase or subscription price.

Letters to the Editor

Letters must be limited to 500 words and should provide thoughtful scientific criticism, rebuttal, or personal data relating to research articles or commentary published in IOTE. No more than five citations and references can be included. Unless specifically indicated to the contrary, all letters will be assumed to be for publication and will be subject to the same editorial revision policies as other manuscripts.

Commentaries

Scholarly discussion of emerging educational issues will be considered.

Submitted manuscripts in this category typically are limited to 2,000 words and must be as succinct, accurate, and informative as possible. In some cases, the Editor may publish a counterpoint or opposing view commentary to stimulate thought and discussion.

Manuscript Submission

Submit manuscripts in *quadruplicate* to the Editor, whose address follows. A cover letter should accompany articles, abstracts, or review manuscripts indicating that the material is not currently under consideration for publication elsewhere. The letter should designate the name of the corresponding author, if different from the senior (first) author.

Authors should retain copies of all material submitted to guard against loss. IOTE cannot assume responsibility for lost manuscripts. If copyrighted material is included in the manuscript, evidence of written permission to reproduce said material must be enclosed with the cover letter. Manuscripts will be acknowledged on receipt. After preliminary review, they will be sent to members of the editorial board. Notification of disposition may take between 2 and 3 months after acknowledgment. Accepted manuscripts will be published only on receipt of signed copyright assignment forms from the authors along with a hard copy and a copy of the entire manuscript on a floppy disk. The copyright so conveyed includes any and all subsidiary forms of publication, including electronic media.

Authors will have the opportunity to review typeset page proofs of the manuscript before publication. Page proofs MUST be returned within 48 hours of receipt—they are for correction only and not for rewrite. Delayed return of page proofs will result in forfeiture of the author's opportunity for prepublication review. IOTE reserves the right to make or request editorial changes in all manuscripts accepted for publication.

Address all editorial correspondence and manuscripts to the Editor, Patricia A. Crist, PhD, OTR/L, FAOTA, IOTE, Department of Occupational Therapy, Rangos School of Health Sciences, Duquesne University, 600 Forbes Avenue, Pittsburgh, Pennsylvania 15282-0020; Internet address (for inquiries or questions only): crist@duq2.cc.duq.edu.

Checklist

(Consult the following instructions before you submit your manuscript package to the American Occupational Therapy Association [AOTA])

1. Print manuscript on one side of standard-sized (8.5 x 11 in. [22 x 28 cm]) white paper.

2. Use either Times Roman or Courier 12-point typeface.

3. Double-space between all lines of the manuscript, including title, headings, footnotes, quotations, references, figure captions, and all parts of tables.

4. Use one space between words. Eliminate all instances of 2 spaces.

5. Leave margins of at least 1 in. (2.54 cm) at the left, right, top, and bottom of every page.

6. Use the flush-left style or ragged right margin of line justification.

7. Indicate a new paragraph by using 2 hard returns, rather than by using tabs or spaces.

8. Turn off the hyphenation function so that no words are divided at the end of the line.

9. Number pages consecutively, beginning with the title page, in the upper right-hand corner.

10. Spell out abbreviations and acronyms the first time they appear in text, follow with abbreviation in parentheses, and use the abbreviation consistently throughout the remainder of the text. Eliminate unnecessary abbreviations.

11. Use generic drug and equipment names; insert proprietary names in parentheses at the point of first mention; if it is necessary to use a trademark, include the manufacturer's name, city, and state.

12. Express weights and measures in standard and metric units; express temperatures in degrees Fahrenheit and in degrees centigrade.

13. Include page numbers in text for all quotations.

14. Cite references in both the text and in the reference list; make sure the entries agree in spelling and in date.

15. Spell out journal titles completely.

16. Alphabetize references in the reference list by the author's surname.

17. Provide inclusive page numbers for all articles or chapters in books.

18. Provide written permission for all materials obtained from other publishers. Include the page numbers of your manuscript to which the permission refers. Provide model releases for any full-face or partial-face photos of persons. Sample release forms are available from AOTA.

19. Provide clearly labeled camera-ready art for all illustrations, including photographs, and mark the locations for placement within the manuscript.

20. Retain a copy of your manuscript, paper files, art, and electronic files. Do not send your only copies.

21. Please understand that your submission is final copy. Pages reviewed later for proofing are for correction only and not for rewrite.

Art Requirements

If possible, submit art on disk and indicate software version used to create information.

Line Drawings, Tables, and Graphs

1. Provide crisp, clean originals in black on smooth white paper.

2. Remove unnecessary smudges.

3. Do not send poor-quality "patchy" photocopies. Be sure photocopies include the complete page and that the page is evenly reproduced.

4. Do not enclose faxes of artwork because these do not reproduce well.

Photographs

1. Send either color or black-and-white photographs.

2. Use either color or black-and-white prints in the largest format possible (4 x 6 in. or 8 x 10 in.).

3. Use color or black-and-white 35-mm slides or transparencies.

Submit a self-addressed, stamped postcard with your manuscript. On the blank side, provide the authors and title of the manuscript you are submitting for review.

Effective and economical use of your word-processing file depends on its being consistently prepared. Please follow the APA guidelines for preparing a manuscript (chapter 4). You are responsible for ensuring that the electronic files on your submitted diskettes exactly match the hardcopy printout of the submitted manuscript.

Final Manuscript Submission Only (accepted for publication)

(If your article is accepted for publication you will have to meet the following additional requirement when submitting your final edited draft to the Editor)

1. Provide clearly labeled diskettes with your name, telephone number, and file names in WordPerfect 5.1 or Microsoft Word on a 3.5-inch high density diskette (1.44–2 MB).

2. Label your envelope with "disk enclosed" to ensure proper handling by post office personnel.

3. Be sure that all earlier versions of your manuscript are deleted from the disk. ▪